# FOAM
# Rolling

Sam Woodworth

Sam Woodworth

# FOAM Rolling

# CONTENTS

## 5 PAIN RELIEF PROGRAMS

## 6 LIFESTYLE PROGRAMS

## 7 SPORTS PROGRAMS

# INTRODUCTION

Imagine your wellness as a bucket, and optimal mobility is a full vessel, the way you're designed to work. But if you're like most, your movement often feels dysfunctional and strained.

Through daily habits, you subject yourself to extremes that imbalance and weaken the muscular system—holes in the bucket. If you have poor balance, limited mobility, pain, and tightness, you can benefit from a foam roller.

For everyone from the active and agile to the sedentary and tense, rollers and other tools can counteract the negative effect of an 8-hour day sitting, a double shift on your feet, or 10 miles logged as you train. Using a foam roller increases flexibility, promotes healing after injury, improves the alignment of your spine, and heightens your body awareness.

Within this book are 60 step-by-step exercises and 26 programs showing you how to use rolling tools to treat the side effects of your occupational or recreational activities.

Don't allow your lifestyle to sabotage your muscles—use this book to plug the holes in your bucket as you restore your body to its healthiest, happiest, most limber state.

# FOAM ROLLING
# BASICS

# WHY USE A ROLLER?

The foam roller is a multi-purpose tool that can benefit just about anyone. Rollers are effective as both deep-tissue massagers and as props to build strength and bring your body into alignment.

Breathing is easier when your muscles are limber

Your spine is longer and more relaxed with frequent rolling

## ROLLING VS. STATIC STRETCHING

Both static stretching and foam rolling increase your range-of-motion. However, holding a static stretch too long and too often can reduce your muscles' ability to contract (shorten). On the other hand, foam rolling increases the flexibility of your muscles while maintaining their healthy ability both to lengthen (stretch) and to contract.

## RELIEVE PAIN

Overworked muscles lead to aching imbalances and trigger points. Using a foam roller to massage your body's soft tissue improves circulation and alleviates pain.

## IMPROVE POSTURE AND ALIGNMENT

Your muscles conform to your lifestyle, causing them to become chronically shortened or lengthened. Rolling restores muscle balance and aligns vertebrae for better posture.

## MORE REASONS TO ROLL

**1** It's inexpensive
Foam rolling requires little investment in equipment or gym memberships and trainers.

**2** You can do it anywhere
Foam rollers are lightweight and easy to store, so use them at home, at the gym, or even outside.

**3** You can go solo
You don't need the assistance of a coach or workout partner—just yourself and some open space.

**4** It's not just for athletes
Rolling can benefit people of all abilities and lifestyles, from desk workers to stay-at-home parents.

**5** It's versatile
Although it's considered a massage tool, also use it to add a challenging element to your fitness routine.

**6** It helps you de-stress
Rolling away the knots and aches helps you relax at the end of a hard day, just like a deep tissue massage.

High-density foam applies pressure to your soft tissue to loosen the muscles

### AID RECOVERY

The damage to muscle fibers after an injury or workout causes muscle tension. Rolling your muscles breaks up scar adhesions, reduces tightness, and accelerates healing.

### INCREASE BODY AWARENESS

Underuse dulls your muscles and sensory input, but regularly using a foam roller for exercise and massage sharpens your body's sense of how it can effectively move in space.

### BUILD STRENGTH

A muscular body is more functional and pain-free. Use your roller as an exercise prop to build core strength. Also challenge and build your arms and legs with massage exercises.

# USING A ROLLER FOR MASSAGE

Habits and lifestyles shape your muscle use and movement, often resulting in pain and dysfunction. Using a roller and other massage tools releases tension in your body's soft tissue and restores proper movement.

## WHY YOUR BODY NEEDS MASSAGE

Occupation, fitness level, and daily habits affect your body's skeletal and neuromuscular system. These structures assimilate to your posture, so whether standing all day or sitting, your bones and soft tissues fix themselves in position. This causes muscle groups to pull on each other, with too much stress on some and not enough on others. The imbalanced system reduces your flexibility and movement quality.

## MYOFASCIA AND MOVEMENT

These muscle imbalances affect your *fascia,* the flexible network of soft tissue that contains and connects every structure in your body. Muscles are specifically bound by *myofascia*. When myofascia is static, it hardens, but with mechanical stress, it is naturally more fluid. Healthy myofascia allows your muscles to slide flexibly and efficiently in your body while staying in place.

However, your myofascia thickens under stress so it can support your posture and muscle imbalances. For example, a pectoral muscle that never reaches full length develops myofascial adhesions to brace the shortened state. This causes the chest muscles to feel taut and inflexible. Hardened myofascia constricts your muscle fibers and leads to poor circulation of blood and oxygen. Restricted muscles limit range-of-motion and make your body tense.

## RESTORATION BY ROLLING

Massaging your muscles with a foam roller and other tools softens your myofascia so that the structures within—contracted muscle fibers—can receive oxygenated blood. This technique is called self-myofascial release (SMR). Massaging the soft tissue breaks up adhesions and returns it to a flexible state. When you practice SMR regularly, it can restore smoothness to your fascia, improve circulation, decrease pain, and increase overall range-of-motion.

### WHAT ARE TRIGGER POINTS?

Trigger points (also called knots) are small, painful spots that form in your muscle fibers. They occur when the portion of the muscle fiber that contracts—called the *sarcomere*—becomes overworked and locked in a shortened state that restricts blood flow. Hundreds of contractions in the same spot of a muscle form a trigger point. Direct massage to a trigger point with a smaller tool (like a lacrosse ball) unlocks the sarcomeres to restore blood flow and reduce pain.

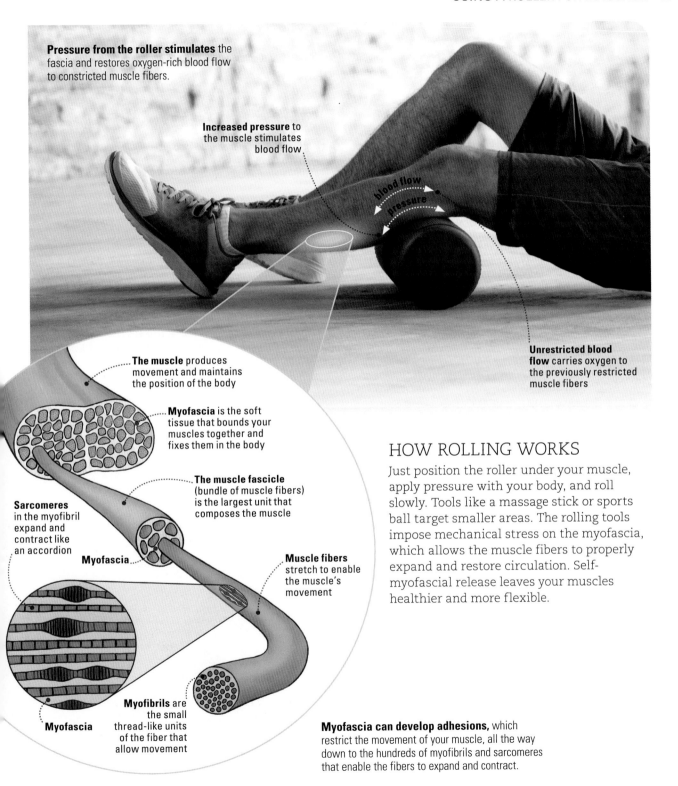

**Pressure from the roller stimulates** the fascia and restores oxygen-rich blood flow to constricted muscle fibers.

**Increased pressure** to the muscle stimulates blood flow

blood flow

pressure

**Unrestricted blood flow** carries oxygen to the previously restricted muscle fibers

**The muscle** produces movement and maintains the position of the body

**Myofascia** is the soft tissue that bounds your muscles together and fixes them in the body

**The muscle fascicle** (bundle of muscle fibers) is the largest unit that composes the muscle

**Sarcomeres** in the myofibril expand and contract like an accordion

**Myofascia**

**Muscle fibers** stretch to enable the muscle's movement

**Myofascia**

**Myofibrils** are the small thread-like units of the fiber that allow movement

## HOW ROLLING WORKS

Just position the roller under your muscle, apply pressure with your body, and roll slowly. Tools like a massage stick or sports ball target smaller areas. The rolling tools impose mechanical stress on the myofascia, which allows the muscle fibers to properly expand and restore circulation. Self-myofascial release leaves your muscles healthier and more flexible.

**Myofascia can develop adhesions,** which restrict the movement of your muscle, all the way down to the hundreds of myofibrils and sarcomeres that enable the fibers to expand and contract.

# MORE FOAM ROLLER BENEFITS

The foam roller can act as a prop and source of feedback for strength training exercises. Exercising with a roller as a prop makes your movement more functional and improves your posture and balance.

## BUILD CORE STRENGTH

The foam roller introduces instability to your exercises, which will intensify the engagement of your core. Working out on a stable surface can eventually become too easy; by adding a foam roller, the instability recruits the whole kinetic chain and deeper-lying muscles to maintain balance. After mastering certain exercises on a stable surface, add a roller so holding the position is more challenging. Remember to keep your lower back static and maintain a neutral spine so your exercises are safe and effective.

## OPTIMIZE BODY AWARENESS

Whether you're minimally active or you're athletic and agile, using a roller improves body awareness, also called *proprioception*. Self-myofascial release exercises awaken and sharpen sensory input, and core-strengthening exercises recruit the kinetic chain to act harmoniously. Together, both types of exercise develop the signals in your muscles that provide information to your brain, asking the body to act deliberately. You'll learn improved positioning relative to the ground, and you will naturally act with balance and improved reaction time.

### YOGA PROP

You can creatively use a foam roller as a prop for several yoga poses. Insert the roller into any pose where you need extra relief to your joints in an uncomfortable position. Or place the roller on the ground and use it for balance.

**Child's Pose**
Use a foam roller for the popular Child's Pose. Place it between your posterior thighs and calves to prevent hyperflexion and discomfort in the knee joints.

**Twisted Dragon**
Modify the Twisted Dragon pose with a foam roller to make the position less extreme. This stretch is a great addition to rotational exercises.

# IMPROVE POSTURE AND ALIGNMENT

Sitting in a car or at a desk all day, looking down at a cell phone screen, and reaching for a keyboard deteriorate a natural and healthy posture. Regularly foam rolling will restore flexibility to your soft tissues so that your muscle groups lengthen and contract as a functional orchestration. Balanced and limber muscles allow your body to achieve a healthy posture and your bones to rest in pain-free alignment.

Also use the roller as a feedback prop to strengthen weaker muscles and lock in good posture. Place the roller just beside the moving body part during certain exercises. If the roller falls or excessively moves, you can determine that stronger, synergist muscles are compensating for weaker muscles. This feedback method teaches your body to work in more optimal orchestration, which aligns the spine and stabilizes your posture.

Strengthen and lengthen your muscles with upper body exercises for healthy movement and proper alignment

Improve the mobility of your ribcage and related joints with rotational exercises

Stabilize your hips in a variety of positions with lower body exercises

Minimize strain and dysfunction of the knee joints by strengthening surrounding muscles

Massage your feet to sharpen sensory input to the brain and improve proprioception

# EFFECTIVE ROLLING

To get the most of your rolling experience, it's important to use the roller safely by employing principles of proper breathing and positioning. It's also critical to maintain awareness of your body's feedback.

## MONITOR YOUR BODY'S RESPONSE

Using a foam roller or other rolling tool for self-myofascial release (SMR) requires attentiveness to your body's response. Foam rolling should elicit a "good" pain, neither excruciating nor effortless. Most exercises recommend 20 to 30 seconds of rolling, but you should listen to your body and massage only as long as the sensation feels good. A release session should leave your muscles relaxed, rejuvenated, and limber.

### PAIN SCALE

Using a roller should produce pain within the 1 to 3 range. Adjust pressure so the exercises are just slightly uncomfortable.

0    1    2    3    4    5

### SMR Rolling Tips

- Keep breathing.
- Don't go too fast.
- Relax your muscles as much as possible.
- Stop rolling if it's too painful.

## GET INTO POSITION

Align your head neutrally with your spine

Sit at the end of the roller and slowly lie back

Minimize the space between your lower back and the roller

**Back-lying**
Lie on the roller for exercises that target your alignment. Your lower and upper back should maintain contact with the roller throughout.

Align your head with your spine

Lift your hips to align them with your head

Allow slight curves in your spine

Plant your foot on the ground

**Side-lying**
You'll vary this position for exercises that target muscles on the side of the body. Use your support forearm and leg to propel movement.

## PRACTICE CONSCIOUS BREATHING

Proper breathing is critical for maintaining a relaxed state, and only relaxed muscles are receptive to self-myofascial release. Deep, conscious breathing enhances your ability to perceive sensations and contractions in particular muscles.

Inhale through your nose during the easier part of a movement

Exhale through your mouth during the harder part of a movement

Expand your ribcage outward rather than upward

Pull upward through the head to elongate your torso

Anchor your ribcage and engage your abdomen

Plant your feet hip-width apart on the ground

Allow slight, neutral curves in your neck and lower back

Align your shoulders over your arms

Maintain a neutral spine with slight curves at the lower back and neck

Keep your elbows soft, or slightly bent

**Sitting**
For exercises that require a chair, be sure to sit at the edge. To get into position, sit on the bony prominence of your rear, then lengthen the torso.

**Kneeling or plank**
Use this position to engage the abdomen for many core exercises. For effective exercises, channel pressure through the support arms.

# WHAT YOU NEED

The exercises in this book don't require lots of expensive or hard-to-find equipment. Choose your tools based on your degree of body awareness, level of pain perception, and overall goals.

## ROLLERS

Foam rollers come in a variety of shapes, sizes, textures, and colors. Texture and density affect the intensity of your release, and the size and shape of a roller make it particularly suited for certain exercises. You'll want to select a roller that can meet a majority of your needs and goals. For basic massage and exercise when you're just starting out, it's best to keep it simple with a circular roller.

You can rest your whole back and head on these longer rollers

### Circular Roller
This is the most common type of roller, available in all sorts of lengths and densities. It's used for most of the exercises in this book.

### Half Roller
The half roller doesn't actually roll, but it's more stable than a circular roller and is a useful prop to stand on in many exercises.

Stand with the curved side to the ground to challenge your balance

### Textured Roller
This advanced foam roller uses texture to provide points of increased pressure on your soft tissue. The extra mechanical stress elicits extra release.

Spikes and ridges deeply penetrate the fascia

## TIP
To choose a beginning roller, consider how to maximize mechanical stress on soft tissue without exceeding your pain tolerance. Try a smooth, 36-inch (92cm) roller.

## ○ CHOOSING THE RIGHT ROLLER

There is no one-size-fits-all foam roller. The best roller for you is one that's comfortable, effective, and not too painful. If you can, test your roller before you buy it.

Consider these factors:

### 1 Shape
Choose a circular roller if you want to release large muscles groups or to perform most core and balance exercises. Use a half roller as an exercise prop if you want to modify exercises in which you're not actually rolling the foam roller.

### 2 Length and diameter
Consider that a longer roller is bulkier but stable and great for back exercises. A shorter roller is harder to control but more portable and best for leg exercises.

Most are 18 or 36 inches (46 or 92cm) long. While they're usually 6 inches (15cm) in diameter, a smaller diameter is great for aging or physical therapy patients.

### 3 Material and density
Determine if your pain tolerance and desired level of release require a more or less dense roller. A standard roller uses high-density foam and provides moderate release, while a plastic core roller (often hollow) provides more intense release.

### 4 Texture
Choose texture based on your level of muscle tension. A roller with bumps and ridges adds additional points of pressure to your soft tissue, which maximizes release. A smooth roller distributes pressure, so the massage is more gentle.

## OTHER TOOLS

Several exercises and modifications in this book incorporate sports balls and massage sticks. They grant additional control and pressure to your exercises, which are especially important for relieving trigger points.

Lacrosse ball

### Sports Balls
Firm sports balls are crucial for trigger point release. They provide a concentrated point of pressure for tense muscles. This book features a lacrosse ball in the targeted release exercises.

Golf ball

Tennis ball

### OTHER EQUIPMENT YOU MAY WANT

**Yoga mat** Many exercises require you to be on the ground, so a nonskid mat increases comfort and safety.

**Chair** Some exercises and modifications are easier if you sit in a chair or rest your hands on it for balance.

**Pillow** Lay on a pillow to relieve neck tension, or place a pillow on the ground to establish easier endpoints for some back-lying rotational exercises.

### Massage Sticks
Massage sticks also provide more targeted release than a foam roller. Since you hold a massage stick with your hands, it's a good way to modify any exercise so that the position and movement is easier.

# BEFORE YOU BEGIN

Before you get started with this book, take some time to consider what your needs are and which programs or exercises best suit you. With the right tools and the right environment, you're ready to get rolling.

## EVALUATE YOUR NEEDS

Everyone engages in repetitive patterns of movement that disrupt the body's alignment and cause muscle tension and pain. Consider your daily habits and areas of pain, and choose the exercises and programs that will benefit you most.

## CHOOSE A PROGRAM

In the last three chapters of the book are 26 programs (each 5 to 10 exercises) that tend to particular needs. Some address work conditions, and others athletic activities. For example, if you play tennis, consider the Rotational Sports program.

| HABIT AND EFFECT | REMEDY |
| --- | --- |
| **Spending all day at a desk** over- and underworks a myriad of muscles within the legs, hips, and spine, which imbalances the whole muscular system. | **Roll the hip flexors, hamstrings, and chest area,** and strengthen your entire backside. Trigger point release may be necessary in the upper back and shoulders. |
| **Driving more than an hour** strains muscles in your upper back and shoulders and shortens the chest muscles, in addition to underworking the legs and hips. | **Release the chest muscles** to reduce tightness, and strengthen the upper back muscles to improve posture. Massage your hip flexors and quadriceps. |
| **Looking down at a phone or tablet** shortens muscles in the front of the neck and the chest and overstretches muscles in the back of the neck and upper back. | **Roll the chest, shoulders, and arms** to reduce tightness. You may also need to address trigger points of the lower arms and hands caused by holding devices. |
| **Frequently reaching overhead** overlengthens the neck and shoulder muscles and strains the lower back, which deteriorates alignment. | **Release the shoulders and upper back,** and choose exercises to lengthen and restore your spine to improve vertebral alignment. |
| **Spending all day on your feet** stiffens your hips and legs, reduces flexibility, and inflames the fascia in the bottom of the feet. | **Massage your feet** and roll the entire lower body to improve range-of-motion in stiff joints. Strengthen the relationship of your core and lower body. |
| **Carrying a heavy bag on your shoulder** creates asymmetry in your shoulder and hip alignment and throws off your natural gait. | **Release your shoulders and core,** especially on the side where you carry the load. Perform rotational exercises to offset asymmetry. |

## FOAM ROLLING Q&A

### How often should I use a roller?
Use a foam roller at least three times per week for the best results. There's no research that too much self-myofascial release is harmful.

### How long should I spend on each exercise?
Usually 20-30 seconds provides adequate release, but roll as long or as short as feels good.

### Using a roller hurts! Am I doing it wrong?
Some discomfort is normal, but don't exceed your pain tolerance. In general, if you can't maintain comfortable breathing, reduce the pressure.

### Can I create my own program?
Yes, modify the programs in this book or create your own to fit your lifestyle or limitations. Determine your primary need, and choose 5 to 10 exercises. For thorough release, foam roll first, then do the targeted release exercises.

### What kind of results can I expect?
If you do the exercises properly and frequently, you can expect less pain, better posture, and enhanced mobility in previously restricted joints. You'll feel better after just one release session, so keep it up.

### When should I use my foam roller?
Roll whenever you have time, but especially before and after a workout. Rolling before you go to bed can give you a more relaxed sleep, and rolling when you wake up primes your body for a productive day.

### Who can benefit from foam rolling?
Anyone from elite athletes to desk workers can benefit from massage.

### Should I do it even if I don't have any issues?
Yes! Prevention plays a critical role in maintaining your muscles, so massage regularly to keep them healthy and flexible.

## COUNTDOWN TO ROLLING

- Use your foam roller in an open space with room to fully extend your arms and legs.
- Pull back long hair and avoid thick, baggy clothing.
- Find a nonskid surface on which to do your exercises.
- Remove your shoes if you plan to stand on the roller or massage your feet.

# CORE
# EXERCISES

# PLANK PROGRESSIONS

Since crunches and sit-ups reinforce rounded posture, the plank is a great way to support an erect stance. This exercise outlines three progressions—advance your plank when you master the previous one with strength and perfect posture.

**TARGETED MUSCLES**

This exercise targets the obliques, the abdomen, and the shoulder blade stabilizers. Strengthening these muscles makes the body more stable and efficient.

FRONT          BACK

**1**

**Lie on your stomach** and place the foam roller beneath your shins. Put your forearms and palms flat on the ground.

**HOW IT HELPS**
Planks strengthen the core to restore posture. The spinal position is often compromised, but engaging the abdomen stabilizes the vertebral column.

Maintain a tense, neutral spine

**2**

**Lift your body** off the ground by pushing through your forearms, and contract your abdomen. Hold for 1 minute.

Keep a neutral spine
and relax your neck

**3**

**Progress to a more difficult plank** by shifting the
roller closer to your feet. Hold for 1 minute.

Keep your hips level

**4**

**Shift the roller down** beneath your toes. Hold the
plank for 1 minute.

Maintain regular
breathing

**5**

**Place the roller beneath your shins** and reach your arms out, one
at a time. Alternate your reach with each arm for 1 minute.

# ROLLER ROLLOUT

Lock in good posture throughout your day by doing the Roller Rollout. This core-strengthening exercise produces a bigger contraction of the abdomen than a traditional sit-up, so it dramatically improves your body's ability to remain in alignment.

**TARGETED MUSCLES**

This exercise targets the core musculature and the *latissimus dorsi* and *teres major* muscles of the back. These influence shoulder position and spinal alignment.

FRONT          BACK

Face your palms to each other

**1**

**Kneel** and place the foam roller in front of you. Position the sides of your hands on the roller, shoulder-width apart.

Inhale as you roll forward

Maintain a neutral spine

**2**

**Roll forward** from the hips, allowing the roller to glide up your hands and forearms.

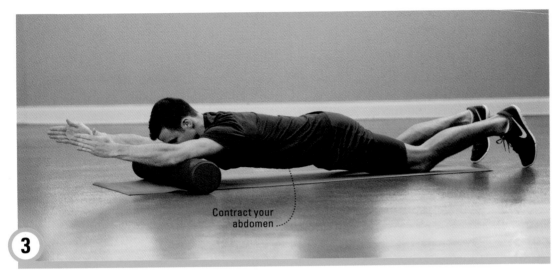

**3**

**Continue to roll** over the foam roller until your arms and hips reach full extension.

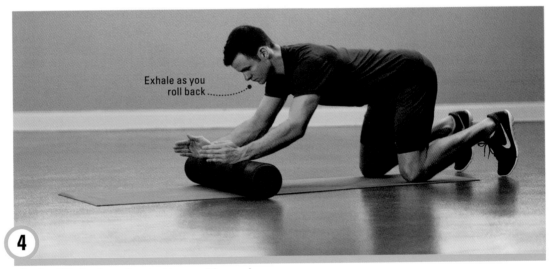

**4**

**Slowly slide back** to the starting position and repeat the exercise 15 times.

## CAUTION
To avoid shoulder or back injury, stop if you feel any pain and regress to a less challenging core exercise, like Plank Progressions.

# ROLLER WALKOUT

This challenging core and shoulder exercise improves torso stability in many positions, like standing upright and sitting. The Roller Walkout translates to better posture and balance during exercise and daily activities by strengthening the core.

**1**

**Place your hands** shoulder-width apart on the foam roller and lift your body into a push-up position. Align your shoulders over your arms.

Straighten your legs, but don't lock your knees

**2**

**Walk your feet in** toward your hands, keeping your legs straight and lifting your hips until they're aligned over your feet.

**TIP**
To improve stability in the shoulder joints, point your middle finger forward and rotate your arms inward as you walk forward.

Maintain a neutral spine

**3**

**Walk your feet back** as far as possible, extending your arms, straightening your legs, and engaging your core.

Relax your neck

Maintain downward pressure through your hands into the roller to engage your core.

**4**

**Walk your feet slightly forward** to return to the starting position. Repeat the exercise 10 times.

# BIRD DOG REACH

Incorporating the foam roller with the Bird Dog Reach provides feedback on your balance and tests your ability to distribute load across one hip and shoulder. It's a great way to develop spine and hip control during one-leg-stance actions, like walking.

## TARGETED MUSCLES

This exercise targets the abdominals, obliques, gluteals, and deltoids, which stabilize the pelvis and torso and improve movement efficiency.

FRONT          BACK

...Look at the ground to avoid neck tension

**1**

**Kneel on all fours** and place the foam roller next to your left hip. Align your shoulders over your hands and your hips over your knees.

**TIP**
To keep excessive pressure off your wrists and to stabilize your torso, channel your weight through the supporting palm and knee.

**2**

**Reach your left arm** straight out in front of you and reach your right leg straight out behind you, trying not to move the roller.

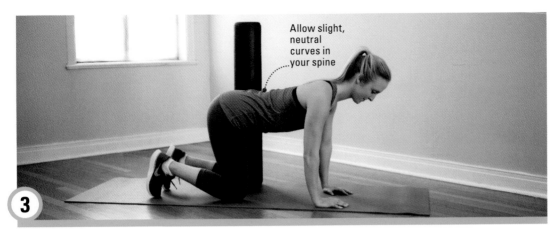

Allow slight,
neutral
curves in
your spine

**3**

**Return your arm and leg** to the starting position,
trying not to move the roller. Repeat the exercise
10 to 15 times with your left arm and right leg.

Lead with
your heel as
you extend
your leg

**4**

**Switch the roller** to your right hip and repeat the
exercise with your right arm and left leg.

## MODIFICATIONS

**To make it easier,** first move just your arm, then progress
to moving just your leg.

**To make it harder,** widen your knees and
hands to challenge your core musculature.

# HIP SWIVEL

For those with limited spine mobility or for rotational sport athletes, this core exercise addresses functional rotation of the pelvis and torso. Using the foam roller activates the hip adductors and challenges your core, integrating them for effective twisting.

**TARGETED MUSCLES**

This exercise targets the obliques of the outer abdomen and the hip adductors of the inner thigh. They support the rib cage and hips.

FRONT          BACK

**1**

**Lie on your back** and extend your arms out from your body, palms facing up. Plant your feet on the ground and place the foam roller between your knees.

Maintain moderate pressure on the roller

**2**

**Raise your legs**, align your knees over your hips, and bend your knees to 90 degrees.

Inhale deeply
through your nose
as you rotate out
to stabilize your
lumbar spine

**3**

**Rotate your hips** and thighs to the left and rotate
your left arm. When your right shoulder begins
to lift off the ground, rotate back to the starting
position. Repeat the exercise 10 times to the left.

**4**

**Repeat the exercise** 10 times to your right.

○ **MODIFICATION**

**To make it easier**,
stack pillows on each
side of your body to
establish easier
endpoints for your
range-of-motion.

**TIP**
For less tension in your
neck, lay your head on
a pillow. Minimal
tension in peripheral
muscles makes the
exercise safer and
more effective.

# SITTING RIBCAGE ROTATION

If you sit for prolonged periods, you'll benefit from this mobility-enhancing exercise. Good range-of-motion in your thoracic spine limits excessive movement in the lower back. Using the roller to activate your adductors helps stabilize the often painful area.

## TARGETED MUSCLES

This exercise targets the thoracic spine, from the neck to the lower back, as well as the abdomen. These areas are responsible for bending and twisting the torso.

FRONT          BACK

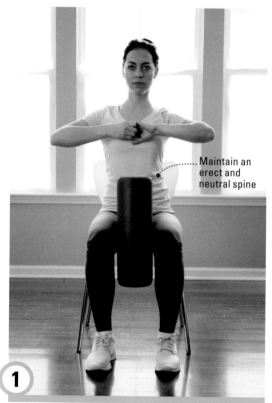

Maintain an erect and neutral spine

**1**

**Sit on the edge of a chair** and place the foam roller between your knees. Clasp your hands together and place them on your sternum. Bend your hips, knees, and ankle joints to 90 degrees.

Exhale through your mouth as you rotate out

Keep tension on the roller throughout the exercise

**2**

**Rotate your arms and torso** to the right until you reach the end of your range-of-motion.

**TIP**
To fix asymmetrical alignment, do more repetitions to one side. For example, golfers or painters may have more tightness in one side than the other.

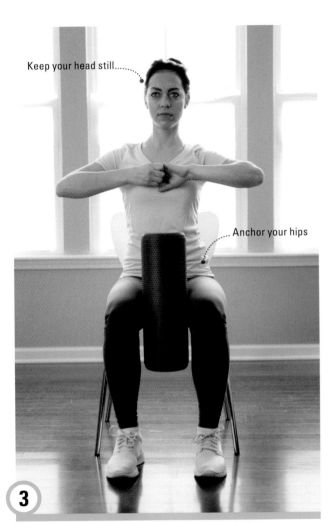

Keep your head still

Anchor your hips

**3**

**Rotate back** to the starting position and repeat the full rotation 20 times to your right side.

Relax your neck

**4**

**Repeat the exercise** 20 times to your left side.

# HALF-KNEELING CORE ROTATION

To mimic everyday mechanics like walking and running, the Half-Kneeling Core Rotation dynamically incorporates the hips with torso rotation. By using a roller for feedback, it indicates whether hip tightness inhibits your rotational performance.

## TARGETED MUSCLES

This exercise targets the core musculature, the gluteal group, and the hip adductor muscles. They help rotate the torso from side to side while walking.

FRONT          BACK

Align your right hip over your right knee.

Align your left knee over your left foot

**1** **Kneel on your right knee** and plant your left foot on the ground. Place the foam roller beside the inside of your left knee and cross your arms over your chest. Inhale to prepare for the movement.

Keep your head still

**2** **Engage your right gluteals,** exhale, and rotate your torso to the left. When you reach the end of your range-of-motion, rotate back to the starting position. Repeat the rotation 10 times to the left.

**TIP**
To improve your ability to do the rotation, also perform release exercises for your lats and gluteal group. Poor flexibility in one muscle group inhibits the other group.

**4**

**Repeat the rotation** 10 times to the right.

Relax your shoulders and neck

Anchor your hips

**3**

**Kneel on your left knee,** switch the roller to the inside of your right knee, and cross your arms.

**MODIFICATION**

**For a different type of feedback,** place the foam roller beside the outside of your support knee.

# SIDE-LYING RIBCAGE ROTATION

The Side-Lying Ribcage Rotation strengthens your ability for thoracic rotation (twisting of the upper and middle back) in relation to your inner thighs. It's a good intermediate challenge if you find the Half-Kneeling Core Rotation too difficult.

**TARGETED MUSCLES**

This exercise targets the adductor muscle group of the inner thighs and the core musculature. These muscles control leverage for torso rotation.

FRONT          BACK

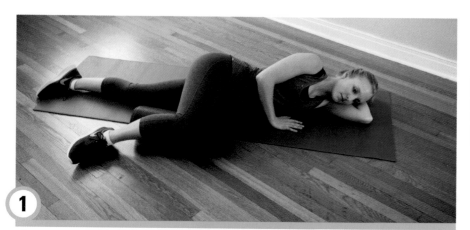

**1**

**Lie on your left side,** straighten your left leg, and bend your right knee and hip to 90 degrees. Place the foam roller beneath your right knee.

**CAUTION**
To avoid muscular strain, do not exceed comfortable range-of-motion. Your level of mobility should determine your degree of rotation.

**2**

**Grasp your ribcage** with your right hand, slightly below your sternum, and inhale.

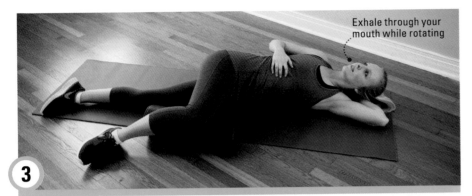

Exhale through your mouth while rotating

**3**

**With your right hand,** pull your torso back as far as possible without allowing your right knee to lift off the roller.

**4**

**Slowly return** to the starting position and repeat the rotation 10 times to the right.

**MODIFICATION**

**5**

**Move the roller** to your left leg, and repeat the rotation 10 times to the left.

**To increase pressure,** use your resting arm and push your knee against the roller for deeper rotation.

# STRAIGHT-LEG RAISE

A great staple for any exercise routine, the Straight-Leg Raise emulates walking and running mechanics. The movement integrates core strength with your ability to stabilize one hip while mobilizing the other, like you do in any single-leg stance.

**TARGETED MUSCLES**

This exercise coordinates movement of the hip flexors, obliques, and abdomen. These are essential for walking.

FRONT        BACK

Bend your ankles to 90 degrees

**1**

**Lie on your back,** relax your arms, straighten your knees, and place your ankles side-by-side on the foam roller.

**TIP**
To take tension off your lower back, engage your core musculature. This allows better mobility in your moving leg.

Exhale as you lift your leg

**2**

**Raise your left leg** straight up, as high as possible without pain or bending your knee. Keep your right leg fixed on the roller.

Inhale as you
lower your leg

**3**

**Lower your left leg** to the starting position and repeat the raise 10
times with your left leg.

**4**

**Repeat the exercise** 10 times with your right leg.

## HOW IT HELPS
Performing this
exercise proficiently
limits hip and lower
back pain. Stability in
one leg while moving
the other is crucial for
healthy mechanics.

## MODIFICATION

**To make it
harder,** raise
both legs, feet
flexed, and
alternate tapping
the roller with
each leg.

# LOWER BODY EXERCISES

# OVERHEAD SQUAT

This more advanced exercise is an excellent full body workout to secure improved posture after a release session. It improves coordination of your muscles from the upper back to the ankles, and the arm component develops overhead mobility.

**TARGETED MUSCLES**

This exercise targets the lower body muscles, the core musculature, and the shoulders. The total body movement strengthens communication of your muscular system.

FRONT        BACK

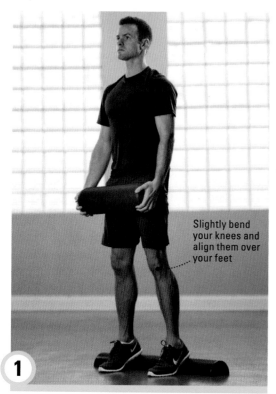

Slightly bend your knees and align them over your feet

**1**

**Stand with your heels** on the curved part of a half foam roller, slightly wider than shoulder-width apart. Hold the ends of a circular roller.

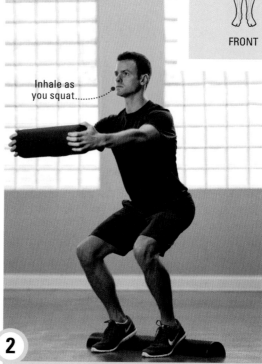

Inhale as you squat

**2**

**Slowly bend at the hips** by sitting your pelvis back and bending your knees. At the same time, begin to raise your arms.

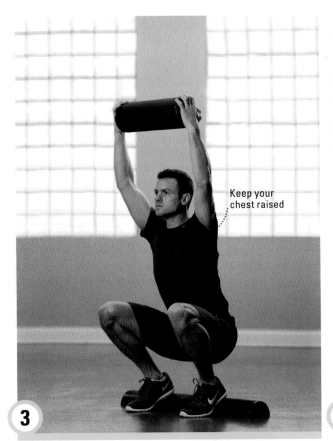

Keep your
chest raised

**3**

**Squat as deeply as possible** and raise your arms until they're straight overhead with your wrists at or behind your head.

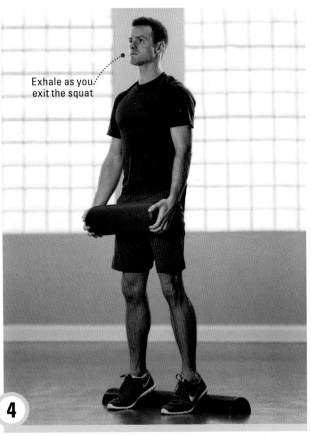

Exhale as you
exit the squat

**4**

**Slowly return** to the starting position and repeat the exercise 15 times.

## MODIFICATIONS

**To make it easier,** cross your arms over your chest if raising them is hard or painful.

**To make it harder,** remove the half roller and plant your feet flat on the ground.

# ROTATIONAL LUNGE

This dynamic exercise is a challenging way to improve the symmetry of your lower body and core muscles. Performing it often is great for any athletic endeavor or lifestyle, as it strengthens and balances the complex orchestration of several muscle groups.

## TARGETED MUSCLES

This exercise targets the gluteal group, quadriceps, hamstrings, and abdomen. Coordination of these muscles is necessary for total movement efficiency.

FRONT          BACK

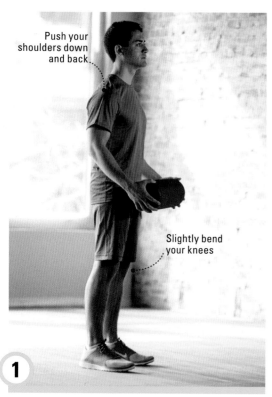

Push your shoulders down and back.

Slightly bend your knees

**1**

**Stand upright,** center your weight over your feet, and hold the ends of the foam roller.

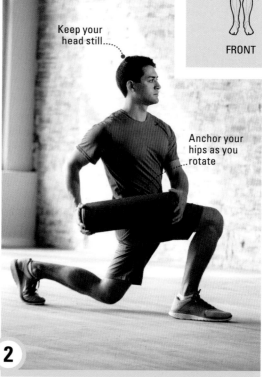

Keep your head still...

Anchor your hips as you rotate

**2**

**Step your right foot forward** and lower your body. As you lunge, rotate your torso to the right and reach the roller around your right leg.

Maintain an erect posture....

Keep tension in your core

**3**

**Press through your left foot,** engage the gluteals, and rotate and step back to the starting position.

**4**

**Repeat the exercise** to your left side. Alternate lunging on each side for a total of 20 repetitions.

## HOW IT HELPS

This exercise improves muscular symmetry. It can help a golfer perform with better balance or a desk worker maintain good posture at work.

○ **MODIFICATION**

**To make it easier,** kneel on one knee and coil and uncoil your torso 10 times to one side, then flip your stance and repeat for the opposite side.

# ADDUCTOR CHAIR SQUAT

This advanced squat is a great full body conditioner. Adding the roller minimizes the distance between your legs and makes the movement more challenging. If you want to lengthen and strengthen your body, then this exercise is a perfect workout addition.

## TARGETED MUSCLES

This exercises targets the deltoids in the shoulder, the abdomen, the gluteal group, the quadriceps, and the *gastrocnemius* muscles in the calves. They're important for movement efficiency and posture.

FRONT          BACK

**1**

Stand upright with your feet shoulder-width apart and point your toes forward.

Face your palms to each other

Squeeze your inner thighs

**2**

Place the foam roller between your thighs. Bend at the hips, sitting your pelvis back and bending your knees. Begin to raise your arms straight up.

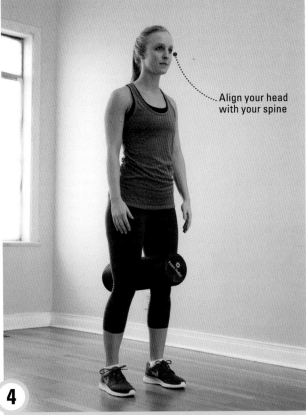

Align your head with your spine

**4**

**Return to the starting position** by lowering your arms, contracting your gluteals, and raising your hips. Repeat the exercise 10 to 15 times.

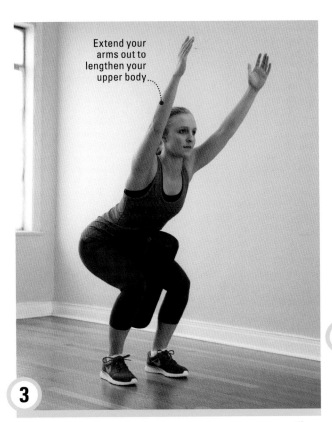

Extend your arms out to lengthen your upper body

**3**

**Squat** to a comfortable depth and raise your arms until they're aligned with your back.

## HOW IT HELPS
This squat balances your knee stabilizers: the hip abductors (outer thighs) and hip adductors (inner thighs). They distribute weight at the hips.

## MODIFICATION

**To make it easier,** place a half roller beneath your heels to allow your hips to descend deeper.

# HIP FLEXOR RELEASE

Hips become easily taut and sensitive when you sit often—in the car, at your desk, or on the couch. Use this exercise to lengthen and restore flexibility to your hip flexors, which tend to be one of the most universally inhibited muscle groups.

## TARGETED MUSCLES

This exercise targets the primary hip flexors, the *psoas* and *iliacus*, which originate in the pelvis and insert in the upper leg. They're responsible for moving the hips.

FRONT          BACK

**1**

**Lie on your stomach** and place the foam roller beneath your left hip. Leave your right leg on the ground and prop yourself up onto your forearms.

## HOW IT HELPS

Releasing tension in the hip flexors alleviates chronic lower back pain by restoring balance to the lower back and pelvic junction.

Rotate your leg in and out while rolling to cover more soft tissue

**2**

**Slowly roll** from your waistline to mid-thigh for 20 to 30 seconds, pushing and pulling with your arms and right leg. Then switch the roller to your right hip and repeat the exercise.

# TARGETED HIP FLEXOR RELEASE

When your hip flexors are shortened, as they are when seated, the muscles receive poor circulation and can develop trigger points. Strenuous running and climbing also contributes to the painful spots. Do this release to restore health to the hip flexors.

**TARGETED MUSCLES**

This exercise targets the primary hip flexors, the *psoas* and *iliacus*, which originate in the pelvis and insert in the upper leg. They assist with standing and walking.

FRONT          BACK

Flatten your torso on the ground

**1**

**Lie on your back** and bend your knees. Place the lacrosse ball on your right hip flexors, halfway between your navel and right hipbone.

Push with your opposite hand and roll the ball in circular motions to massage your hip flexors.

**2**

**Lower your right knee** and roll the ball over your hip flexors for 20 to 30 seconds. Then lower your left knee and repeat the exercise on the left hip flexors.

**TIP**

If your hips are tight and inflexible, place a few pillows beneath your knee to create a comfortable lift.

# TARGETED HIP ROTATOR RELEASE

The *piriformis* is a small hip rotator buried beneath the gluteal group. It's easily inflamed by extensive sitting or standing, causing the muscle to compress the sciatic nerve. Trigger points in this muscle are debilitating, so massaging it is vital for your health.

**TARGETED MUSCLES**

This exercise targets the *piriformis*, a small muscle located beneath the gluteal group. It laterally rotates and abducts the femur in various hip positions.

FRONT          BACK

Rotate your pelvis to the right to increase pressure

**1**

**Sit on the ground** and place the lacrosse ball beneath your left gluteals. Cross your left ankle over your right knee.

Move your left leg side-to-side to adjust pressure on the ball

**2**

**Roll the ball back** to the area above your gluteals, pushing with your arms.

Pressure can aggravate the *piriformis*. Try sitting on a slightly cushioned surface to alleviate pain.

**3**

**Roll the ball forward** to the center of the gluteals. Continue to roll the length of the left *piriformis* for 20 to 30 seconds.

**4**

**Switch the lacrosse ball** to your right gluteals and repeat the exercise.

**TIP**
To alleviate sciatic nerve pressure after you've released trigger points in the *piriformis*, strengthen the muscle. Try the Clamshell Hip Rotation.

**MODIFICATION**

**To decrease pressure,** bend the targeted leg and place the ball beneath the gluteals.

# HIP ROTATOR RAISE

To ensure safe lower extremity movement, this exercise activates the deeper muscles of the hip. These rotate your hips so you don't fall over when walking, but their inactivity leads to problems such as sciatica and overworked peripheral muscles.

**TARGETED MUSCLES**

This exercise targets the *piriformis*, a deep rotator muscle of the hip that lies underneath the gluteal group. It laterally rotates and stabilizes the hip joint.

FRONT          BACK

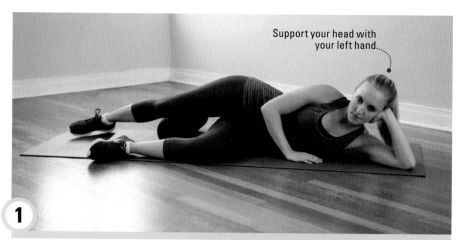

Support your head with your left hand

**1**

**Lie on your left side,** straighten your right leg, and place the foam roller beneath your right knee. Bend your left knee and hip to 90 degrees.

Lead with your heel

**2**

**Anchor your left thigh** and knee in position and slowly rotate your left leg up from the hip until it reaches maximum rotation.

The greater your rotation, the deeper your activation of the hip rotators.

**3**

**Slowly lower your left leg** to the starting position and repeat the exercise 10 to 15 times.

**4**

**Roll over and repeat** the exercise 10 to 15 times for your right hip rotator.

## MODIFICATION

**To make it easier,** sit on the edge of a chair and rotate your leg in front of you to allow more latitude.

### TIP

To maximize the deep contraction of the hip, relax the peripheral muscles. Contracting a small muscle like the piriformis is difficult if larger muscles are also active.

# CLAMSHELL HIP ROTATION

This exercise strengthens the outer thighs to limit your susceptibility to injury and to combat leg ailments like runner's knee. Activate your muscles with this rotation before a workout to keep the knee joints properly aligned with the ankles and hips.

## TARGETED MUSCLES

This exercise targets the *gluteus medius* and *tensor fascia latae*, the hip abductors that originate in the pelvis and insert in the leg. They stabilize the knee and pelvis and pull the leg outward.

FRONT          BACK

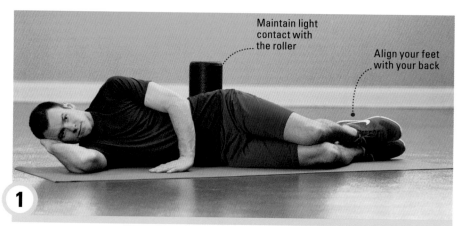

Maintain light contact with the roller

Align your feet with your back

**1**

**Lie on your right side,** stack your legs, and bend your knees to 90 degrees. Place the foam roller behind your pelvis.

## HOW IT HELPS
Strengthening your gluteals ensures that your pelvis is stable when you activate the hips. This prevents injury and eases lower back pain.

Exhale on the upward movement

**2**

**Raise your left knee** as high as you can and hold it for 1 second. Keep your torso still.

Inhale on the downward movement

If the roller moves, then your stronger muscles are compensating for weaker hips.

**3**

**Return your leg** to the starting position and repeat the exercise 15 times with your left leg.

**4**

**Roll over and repeat** the exercise 15 times with your right leg.

**TIP**
To make it harder, ask a partner to apply pressure with his or her hands to the outside of your moving knee during the movement.

# GLUTEAL GROUP RELEASE

If you sit often, then your gluteals—the muscles that keep you upright from the hips—are likely underused. Rolling this area restores hip flexibility to stabilize your lower back and knees. It's a great addition to a warm-up routine before working out.

## TARGETED MUSCLES

This exercise targets the *gluteus maximus*, *medius*, and *minimus*, which are located at the backside of the pelvis. The gluteal muscles keep the body upright.

FRONT          BACK

**1**

**Sit on the foam roller** and place both hands on the ground behind you to hold yourself upright. Extend your legs.

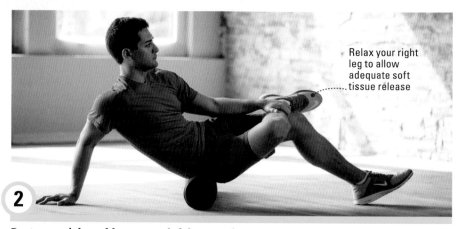

Relax your right leg to allow adequate soft tissue release

**2**

**Rest your right ankle** on your left knee and shift your weight to the gluteals of the right leg. Bend your left knee to increase pressure.

## HOW IT HELPS

This exercise relieves pain from sciatica, a disorder caused by excessive pressure on the sciatic nerve, which runs beneath the gluteal group.

Breathe deeply
to relax your
body

Your gluteal muscles
should melt over the
top of the roller for a
thorough release.

**3**

**Roll back** to your waistline,
pushing with your right arm
and pulling with your left foot.

**4**

**Roll forward** to the top of your thigh. Continue
to roll back and forth over the length of the
right gluteals for 20 to 30 seconds.

**5**

**Uncross your legs and repeat** the exercise for
your left gluteals.

# TARGETED GLUTEAL GROUP RELEASE

Many movements (or a lack of movement) can cause trigger points throughout your gluteal group. While foam rolling the gluteals restores flexibility, using a lacrosse ball to address trigger points makes the muscles more healthy and pain free.

## TARGETED MUSCLES

This exercises targets the *gluteus maximus* and *gluteus medius*. They keep the body upright from the hip and help stabilize the pelvis.

FRONT    BACK

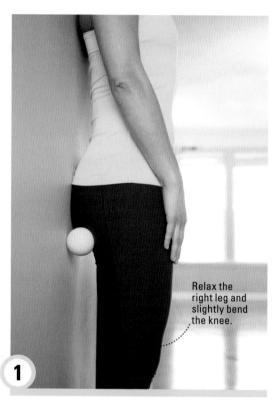

Relax the right leg and slightly bend the knee.

**1**

**Stand upright** and pin the lacrosse ball between the wall and the thickest point of your right gluteals. Lean into the ball.

Use moderate pressure and move your torso in circles to dissolve the trigger points.

**2**

**Bend your knees** to roll the ball over the gluteals. If you find a painful point, massage it with circular movements for 20 to 30 seconds.

**3**

**Rotate your pelvis** to the right and refocus pressure on your outer right gluteals. Roll your muscles over the ball, and spend 20 to 30 seconds massaging particularly painful points.

**4**

**Switch the lacrosse ball** to your left gluteals and repeat the exercise.

### TIP
To avoid underworking the *gluteus medius*, break up long periods of sitting with small walks. Sitting restricts circulation to the gluteals and causes trigger points.

## MODIFICATION

**To increase pressure,** sit on the ground and place the lacrosse beneath your gluteals.

# GLUTEAL BRIDGE

Because the gluteals are commonly underworked, the Gluteal Bridge strengthens the muscles and restores balance to surrounding tissue. If you sit in your car or at your desk a lot, the exercise can significantly improve your movement quality.

## TARGETED MUSCLES

This exercise targets the three muscles of the gluteal group and the hamstrings. Together, they generate massive power for activities like standing up from a seated position or climbing stairs.

FRONT          BACK

**1**

**Lie on your back** and lay your arms at your sides. Put your feet hip-width apart on the foam roller and bend your knees to 90 degrees.

**CAUTION**
To avoid straining your lower back, create outward pressure in your lower abdomen and maintain the slight, neutral curves in your spine.

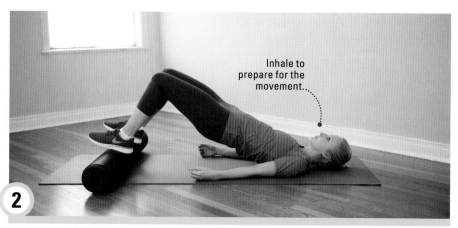

Inhale to prepare for the movement...

**2**

**Raise your hips** until they're aligned with your thighs and you feel your gluteals contract.

Exhale while you
extend your leg....

**3**

**Keep your hips raised** and
extend your left leg out in a
straight line.

Inhale while you
return your leg....

**4**

**Return your left leg** to the foam roller and
extend your right leg, keeping your hips raised.

**5**

**Return your right leg** to the roller and lower your
hips to the starting position. Repeat the exercise
10 to 15 times, or until your muscles fatigue.

 **MODIFICATION**

**To make it harder,** hold the roller
between your knees and squeeze
your inner thigh muscles.

# STRAIGHT-LEG GLUTEAL BRIDGE

Sometimes hip stability and leg mobility are weak and asymmetrical. To make activities like running more efficient, this exercise strengthens your hips, core, and hamstrings to prepare you for single-leg stances and lateral movements.

## TARGETED MUSCLES

This exercise targets the gluteal group, hamstrings, and abdomen. They stabilize the pelvis and enable hip mobility.

FRONT          BACK

Lay your arms at your sides and face your palms down.

**1**

**Lie on your back** and place the foam roller beneath your ankles. Straighten your legs and point your toes upward.

Slightly bend your knee.

Engage your core to protect your spine.

**CAUTION**
To avoid straining your lower back, do not use it to propel the exercise. As a preventative measure, push your lower back into the ground.

**2**

**Raise your left leg** until you feel a stretch in the back of your left hamstrings.

Don't allow your right leg to rotate out during the movement...

**3** Contract your right gluteals and lift your hips 3 to 6 inches (7.5-15.25cm) off the ground.

**4** After 2 seconds, lower your hips and leg.
Repeat the exercise 10 times with your left leg.

**5** Repeat the exercise 10 times with your right leg.

**MODIFICATION**

**To make it easier,** bend your knee to 90 degrees if the hamstrings of your raised leg are too tight.

# QUADRICEPS RELEASE

Rolling your quadriceps is a quick way to improve knee and lower back health. Flexible knee joints allow the hamstrings to fully contract, which in turn balances tension in surrounding areas. This release is great after a long day of driving or sitting.

## TARGETED MUSCLES

This exercise targets the four muscles that compose the quadriceps, which originate at the hip and insert at the knee. They extend the knee and flex the hip.

FRONT          BACK

**1**

Lie on your stomach and place the foam roller beneath your left thigh. Leave your right leg on the ground and prop yourself up onto your forearms.

## HOW IT HELPS
Massaging the quadriceps balances overworked muscles in the entire leg. It loosens the knee joint, allowing full hamstring contraction.

Rotate your leg in and out while rolling to release more soft tissue.

**2**

Roll down to your knee, pulling with your arms and your right leg.

**3**

**Roll up** to the top of your thigh. Continue to roll the length of the quadriceps for 30 to 40 seconds.

**4**

**Switch the foam roller** to your right quadriceps and repeat the exercise.

## MODIFICATIONS

**To make it easier,** sit in a chair and use a massage stick to roll your quadriceps.

**To decrease pressure,** put both legs side-by-side on the roller.

# TARGETED QUADRICEPS RELEASE

The quadriceps muscle group is large and powerful, and trigger points here can lead to pain around the knee and hips. It's great to do this exercise frequently because releasing the quadriceps can significantly alleviate pain in your lower body.

**TARGETED MUSCLES**

This exercise targets the four heads of the quadriceps muscle group in the front thigh: the *rectus femoris*, *vastus lateralis*, *vastus intermedius*, and *vastus medialis*. They contribute to knee extension.

FRONT          BACK

Relax your knee to keep tension off the quadriceps.

**1**

**Slightly bend your right knee** and pin the lacrosse ball between the wall and the middle of your right quadriceps. Lean into the ball.

Rotate your leg in and out to access different trigger points.

Use moderate, sustained pressure and circular movement to dissolve any trigger points.

**2**

**Bend your knees** to roll the ball up to your hip. If you find a painful point, massage it with circular movements for 20 to 30 seconds.

If you have trouble rolling the ball, reposition it with your hand.

**3**

**Straighten your knees** to roll the ball down to your knee, and spend 20 to 30 seconds massaging particularly painful points.

**4**

**Switch the lacrosse ball** to your left leg and repeat the exercise for your left quadriceps.

## HOW IT HELPS
Because the *rectus femoris* contributes to bending the hip, this exercise helps people who sit all day and have referred pain and trigger points.

## MODIFICATION

**To increase pressure,** lie on the ground and place the lacrosse ball beneath the quadriceps.

# OUTER THIGH AND HIP RELEASE

This is one of the most popular foam rolling exercises because it releases the often overworked outer thigh. The massage targets the primary lateral stabilizers of the knee joint, which can be tight because of inactive hip and thigh adductors.

## TARGETED MUSCLES

This exercise targets the *tensor fascia latae* (TFL) muscle, which is continuous with the *iliotibial/*(IT) band, a ligament that runs down the outside of the thigh. They stabilize the pelvis and the knee.

FRONT          BACK

Place as much pressure as tolerable on the hip's soft tissue.

**1**

Lie on your left side and place the foam roller beneath your left hip. Plant your right foot on the ground and prop yourself up onto your left forearm.

**TIP**
To make the exercise easier and more comfortable, sit in a chair, rest your feet on the ground, and roll the area with a massage stick.

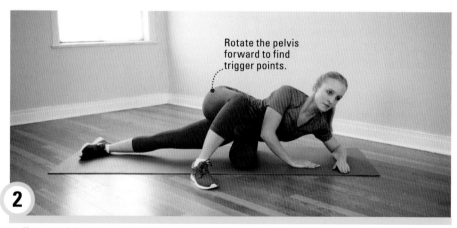

Rotate the pelvis forward to find trigger points.

**2**

Roll up and down on the roller for 20 to 30 seconds between the bony prominences of the hip and pelvis bones. Then switch the roller to your right hip and repeat the exercise.

# TARGETED OUTER HIP RELEASE

This targeted trigger point exercise directly releases points of tenderness in the hip, especially for athletes. Alleviating this area lengthens the IT band, which runs down the outside of your upper leg. Perform this release to improve total leg circulation.

## TARGETED MUSCLES

This exercise targets the *tensor fascia latae* (TFL), an outer hip muscle, and the *gluteus medius*, an outer buttocks muscle. They stabilize lateral knee movement.

FRONT        BACK

**1**

**Stand upright** and pin the lacrosse ball between the wall and the soft tissues of your right hip. Lean into the ball.

**2**

**Bend your right knee** to roll up and down over the hip for 20 to 30 seconds. Then repeat the exercise on your left hip.

Massage the hip with moderate, sustained pressure and circular movements until pain dissipates.

# HAMSTRINGS RELEASE

Muscles are the most efficient when you use them at many lengths, so if you're sitting or standing all day with inactive knees and hips, then your hamstrings are likely tight. Rolling out this tension relieves referred lower back and knee pain.

## TARGETED MUSCLES

This exercise targets the three muscles that compose the hamstrings, located at the back of the thigh. They bend the knee and extend the hip.

FRONT          BACK

**1**

**Sit on the ground** and place the foam roller beneath your right hamstrings. Cross your left ankle over your right ankle.

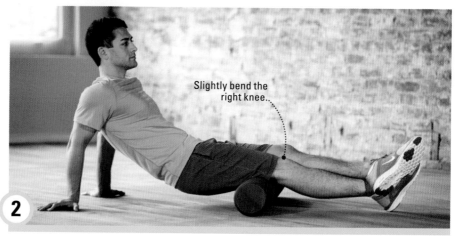

Slightly bend the right knee..

**2**

**Lift your hips** and roll up to your rear, pushing with your arms.

**TIP**
So your hamstrings are receptive to self-myofascial release, relax your feet and maintain deep, conscious breathing.

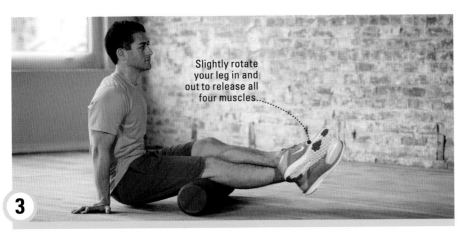

Slightly rotate your leg in and out to release all four muscles...

**3**

**Roll down** to your right knee. Continue rolling the length of the hamstrings for 30 to 40 seconds.

The hamstrings require immense pressure to release, so push your weight down into the roller.

**4**

**Switch the foam roller** to your left hamstrings and repeat the exercise.

## MODIFICATIONS

**To make it easier,** place your foot on a chair and use a massage stick to roll your hamstrings.

**To decrease pressure,** uncross your ankles and roll both legs at the same time.

# TARGETED HAMSTRINGS RELEASE

Releasing hamstrings trigger points starts a beneficial chain reaction that improves total body health. This exercise alleviates pain in the knee and in the back of the thigh. It can even heal headaches and referred pain in your neck caused by short, taut hamstrings.

## TARGETED MUSCLES

This exercise targets the three muscles of the hamstrings: the *biceps femoris*, *semitendinosus*, and *semimembranosus*. They create hip flexion and extension.

FRONT          BACK

Relax your right foot

**1**

**Sit in a chair** and place the lacrosse ball beneath your right thigh. Bend your right knee to 90 degrees and hold the sides of the chair.

On trigger points, move your thigh in a circular motion until you have restored circulation and dissolved pain.

**2**

**Roll the ball back** to your rear by sliding forward. If you find a painful point, massage it with circular movements for 20 to 30 seconds.

**4**

**Switch the ball** to your left thigh and repeat the exercise for your left hamstrings.

**3**

**Roll the ball forward** to your knee by sliding back in the chair, and spend 20 to 30 seconds massaging particularly painful points.

## TIP
To increase pressure on a trigger point, grasp the sides of the chair and pull yourself into the ball. Moderate pressure is best to dissolve these painful spots.

# INNER THIGH RELEASE

This exercise activates the deep muscles of the hip to ensure safe lower extremity movement. Your inner thighs rotate the hips so you stay erect when walking, but their inactivity leads to problems like sciatica and other overworked muscles.

**TARGETED MUSCLES**

This exercise targets the adductor muscle group, which runs from the top of the inner thigh to the inside of the knee. These muscles laterally stabilize the knee joint and help stabilize the pelvis.

FRONT        BACK

**1**

**Lie on your stomach,** prop yourself up onto your forearms, and bend the left hip and knee to 90 degrees. Place the foam roller beneath your left thigh.

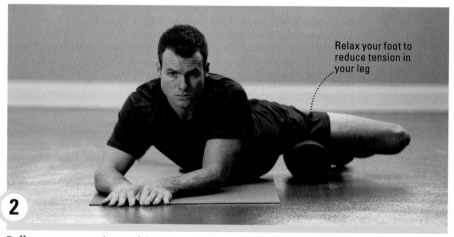

Relax your foot to reduce tension in your leg

**2**

**Roll up** to your groin, pushing yourself to the left with your arms and right leg.

Rotate your pelvis forward and backward to adjust for pressure and comfort

Keep the roller on soft tissue only and avoid rolling your knee joint.

**3**

**Roll down** to your knee. Continue rolling the length of the inner thigh for 20 to 30 seconds.

**4**

**Switch the foam roller** to your right inner thigh and repeat the exercise.

## MODIFICATION

**To make it easier,** sit in a chair, cross your ankle over your knee to access the inner thigh, and use a massage stick to roll the muscles.

**HOW IT HELPS**

Rolling the inner thigh reduces tightness in the outer thigh. Self-myofascial release balances muscle groups that pull on each other.

# TARGETED INNER THIGH RELEASE

Single-leg-stance movements like walking, running, skating, and skiing demand a lot of the inner thighs. The inhibited muscles are often left untreated for trigger points, but massaging them is important for releasing tension in the overused area.

## TARGETED MUSCLES

This exercise targets the *adductor longus*, *adductor brevis*, and *adductor magnus*, the inner thigh hip muscles. They pull the legs toward the body's midline.

FRONT          BACK

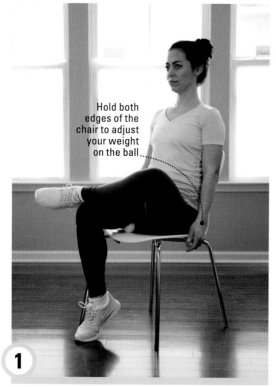

Hold both edges of the chair to adjust your weight on the ball

**1**

**Sit in a chair** and place the lacrosse ball beneath your right inner thigh. Cross your left ankle over your knee and maintain weight on your right leg.

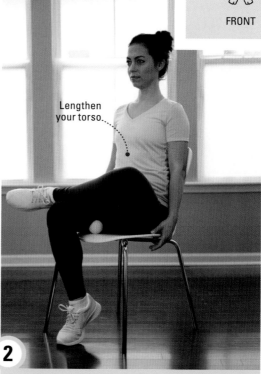

Lengthen your torso

**2**

**Roll the ball forward** to your knee by sliding backward. If you find a painful point, massage it with circular movements for about 25 seconds.

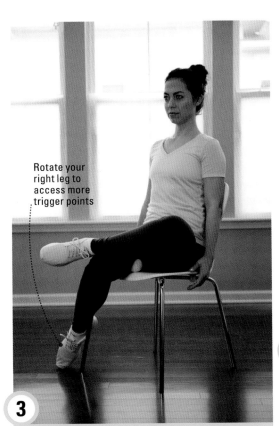

Rotate your right leg to access more trigger points

**3**

**Roll the ball back** to your rear by sliding forward. Spend 20 to 30 seconds massaging painful points.

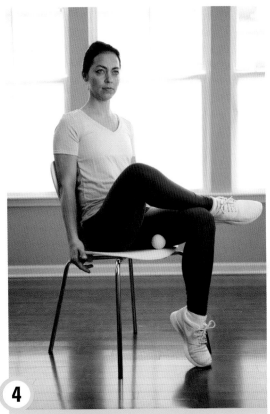

**4**

**Switch the lacrosse ball** to your left inner thigh and repeat the exercise.

## HOW IT HELPS
This exercise releases trigger points caused by a forceful slip. Your inner thighs rapidly activate to stop a fall, but a fast reaction can strain the muscles.

## MODIFICATION

**To decrease pressure,** use your opposite hand to press the lacrosse ball into your inner thigh.

# KNEE RELEASE

The small movement of this exercise releases tension in the knee joint, which becomes strained when you sit or stand all day. It's especially beneficial before any lower body workouts so your leg muscles are flexible and less prone to injuries.

**TARGETED MUSCLES**

This exercise targets the *popliteus* muscle located at the back of the knee. It helps rotate the lower leg and aids other knee movements.

FRONT          BACK

**1**

**Sit on the ground**, place the foam roller beneath your right knee, and plant your left foot on the ground for support.

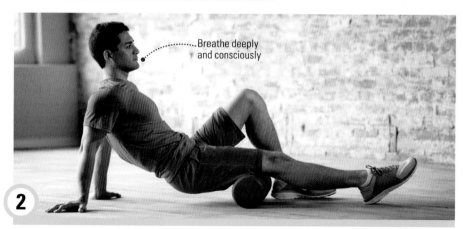

Breathe deeply and consciously

**2**

**Lift your hips** and slightly bend your right knee. Roll up to your thigh, pushing with your arms and pulling with your left foot.

**HOW IT HELPS**
Releasing the knee joint helps the major leg muscles function properly. The *popliteus* assists several muscles during exercise, but it's easily overworked.

Focus pressure on
the soft tissues
under your knee,
never the bones

**3**

**Roll down** to the top of your calf. Continue rolling
the length of your knee for 20 to 30 seconds.

**4**

**Switch the foam roller** to your left knee and
repeat the exercise.

## ◯ MODIFICATIONS

**To increase pressure,** cross your ankles and shift
your weight to the targeted soft tissues.

**For more targeted pressure,** use a lacrosse ball
to pinpoint the small muscle.

# SHIN RELEASE

Easily overused by repetitive movement on hard surfaces, the muscles around your shin bone can become tense and painful. Massage the shin muscles before lower body impact activities to improve the way your legs absorb the vibrations.

**TARGETED MUSCLES**

This exercise targets the *tibialis anterior* and the *extensor digitorum longus* muscles, both located next to the tibia (shin bone). They control several foot movements.

FRONT          BACK

Rotate your left leg out to place pressure on the soft tissue next to the tibia

**1**

**Lie on your stomach,** place the foam roller beneath your left shin, and put your right knee out to the side for leverage. Prop yourself up onto your forearms.

Push your forearms into the ground to activate the core

Minimize direct contact with the tibia

**2**

**Roll up** to the bottom of your knee, pushing with your arms and your right knee.

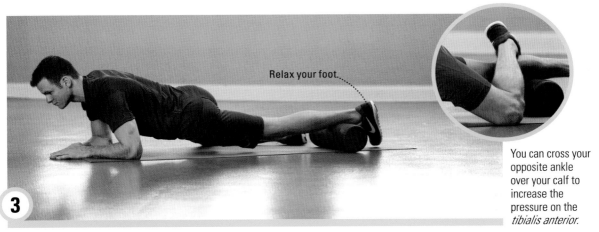

Relax your foot.

You can cross your opposite ankle over your calf to increase the pressure on the *tibialis anterior.*

**3**

**Roll down** to your ankle. Continue to roll the length of the shin for 20 to 30 seconds.

**4**

**Switch the foam roller** to your right leg and repeat the exercise.

**TIP**
To dampen pain from shin splints, release the *tibialis anterior* frequently. Runners and cyclists are often victims of this inflamed muscle, exacerbating the pain.

**MODIFICATION**

**To increase pressure,** cross your feet and focus your weight onto one leg.

# TARGETED SHIN RELEASE

If you're frequently moving on uneven surfaces, the front of your lower legs may be laden with trigger points, which refer pain to your feet. Perform this exercise to release the pain and tension around the shins, big toes, and calves.

**TARGETED MUSCLES**

This exercise targets the *tibialis anterior*, located at the outer side of the tibia (shin bone). It controls several movements of the foot.

FRONT          BACK

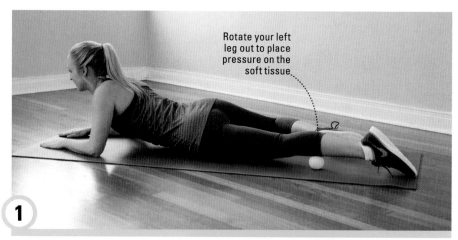

Rotate your left leg out to place pressure on the soft tissue

**1**

**Lie on your stomach** and place the lacrosse ball beneath your left shin. Put your right knee out to the side for leverage.

Relax your left leg so the ball can penetrate the muscle

**2**

**Roll the ball up** to your knee, pushing with your arms and your right knee. If you find a particularly painful point, massage it with circular movements for 20 to 30 seconds.

Relax your foot.

**3**

Rotate your foot to lessen pressure on the shin bone, and use sustained, circular motions to heal trigger points.

**Roll the ball down** to the ankle, and spend 20 to 30 seconds massaging painful points.

**4**

**Switch the lacrosse ball** to your right lower leg and repeat the exercise.

**CAUTION**
To avoid irritating already inflamed soft tissue, don't place too much pressure too soon on the muscle. Gradually increase pressure each time.

**MODIFICATION**

**To make it easier,** sit in a chair and use your heel to penetrate any trigger points.

# CALF MASSAGE

With many occupational hazards, the calf muscles can become overused, tight, and unresponsive, but this exercise restores them to proper function. Roll the area before lower body workouts, especially ballistic exercises that involve jumping.

## TARGETED MUSCLES

This exercise targets the *tibialis posterior*, *gastrocnemius*, and *soleus*, the calf muscles. They control movements of the foot, like pointing the toes.

FRONT          BACK

**1**

**Sit on the ground,** place the foam roller beneath your right calf, and plant your left foot on the ground for support.

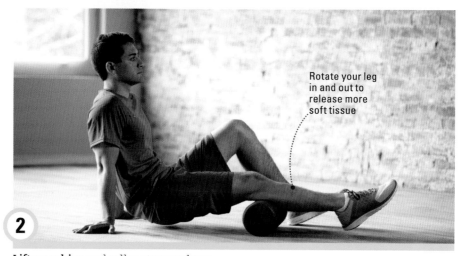

Rotate your leg in and out to release more soft tissue

**2**

**Lift your hips** and roll up to your knee, pushing with your arms and left foot.

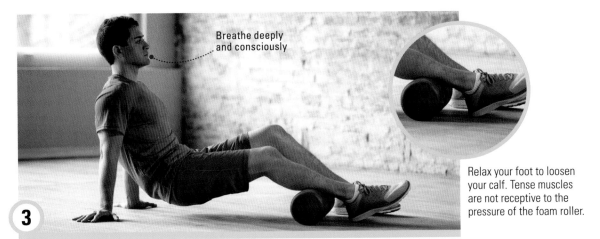

Breathe deeply and consciously

Relax your foot to loosen your calf. Tense muscles are not receptive to the pressure of the foam roller.

**3** **Roll down** to your ankle. Continue rolling up and down the length of the calf for 20 to 30 seconds.

**HOW IT HELPS**
Massaging the calves improves their ability to absorb impact and dampen vibrations. This reduces the chance of shin splints.

**4** **Switch the foam roller** to your left calf and repeat the exercise.

## ⭕ MODIFICATIONS

**To make it easier,** place your foot on a chair and use a massage stick.

**To decrease pressure,** put both legs side-by-side on the roller.

**To increase pressure,** stack your legs and shift your weight to the targeted calf.

# TARGETED CALF RELEASE

This more targeted method releases trigger points in your calf. If you spend all day on your feet, you're a likely victim of the painful spots, but concentrating the pressure can relieve discomfort. It also helps reduce referred pain in the ankles and feet.

**TARGETED MUSCLES**

This exercise targets the *gastrocnemius* and the *soleus* muscles in the calf. They're the primary flexors of the ankle.

FRONT        BACK

**1**

**Sit on the ground** and place the lacrosse ball beneath your left calf. Plant your right foot on the ground for support.

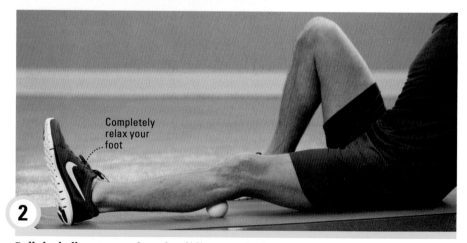

Completely relax your foot

**2**

**Roll the ball up** to your knee by sliding your body forward. If you find a painful point, massage it with circular movements for 20 to 30 seconds.

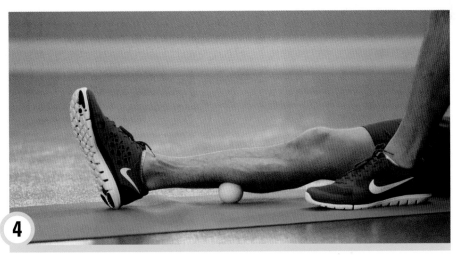

**3**

**Roll the ball down** to your ankle, and spend 20 to 30 seconds massaging painful points.

You may have to use a lot of pressure, so push your calf deeply into the ball to restore blood flow.

**4**

**Switch the lacrosse ball** to your right calf and repeat the exercise.

## HOW IT HELPS
Massaging the calves can relieve cramps. Trigger points do not always actively produce pain, but they can nevertheless cause sporadic spasms.

### MODIFICATION

**To make it easier,** use a massage stick and roll the tool against the trigger points in your calves.

# SPIRAL CALF RAISE

While your feet roll in and out, your hips rotate internally and externally, like when walking. The Spiral Calf Raise develops this relationship so your gait is more proficient, making you less prone to injury during activities that require a spiral movement.

## TARGETED MUSCLES

This exercise targets the *posterior* and *anterior tibialis* (located deep within the lower leg), and the external hip rotators. They control the leg while walking.

FRONT          BACK

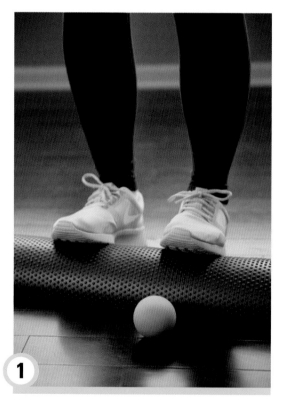

**1**

Stand with the balls of your feet 2 to 4 inches (5-10cm) apart on a half foam roller.

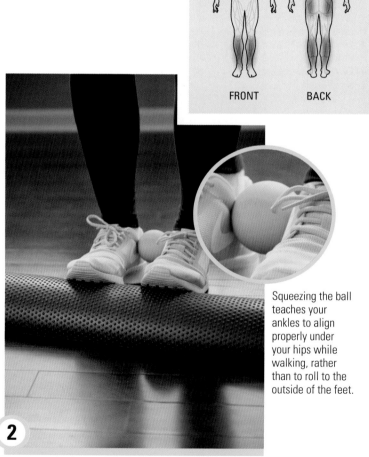

Squeezing the ball teaches your ankles to align properly under your hips while walking, rather than to roll to the outside of the feet.

**2**

Squeeze the lacrosse ball between your heels, just beneath the bones of your ankle joints.

**4**

**After fully contracting your calves,** relax your gluteals and slowly descend back to the starting position. Repeat the exercise 15 times.

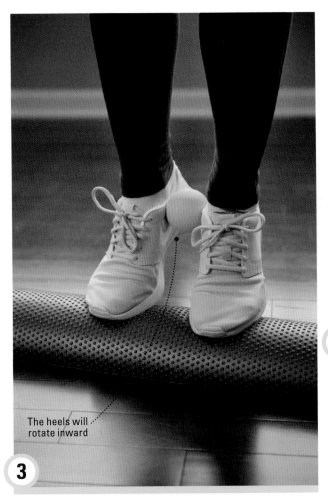

The heels will
rotate inward

**3**

**Push up through your toes** to raise your body with the calf muscles. Simultaneously squeeze your gluteals to rotate your legs externally.

**TIP**

If it's difficult to balance, lightly rest your hands on a wall or chair for support or remove your shoes. Center your weight over your feet.

# ANKLE RELEASE

Use this exercise to relieve tension in your primary ankle-stabilizing muscles, the peroneals. They're often overworked if you walk or run on challenging surfaces, like trails and sand, so roll them before your workout to achieve functional movement.

## TARGETED MUSCLES

This exercise targets the *peroneus longus, brevis,* and *tertius* (the peroneals) located in the outer side of the lower leg. They control several movements of the foot.

FRONT          BACK

Relax your left foot

Channel pressure through your forearm

**1**

**Lie on your left side** and place the foam roller beneath your lower left leg. Plant your right foot on the ground and prop yourself up onto your forearm.

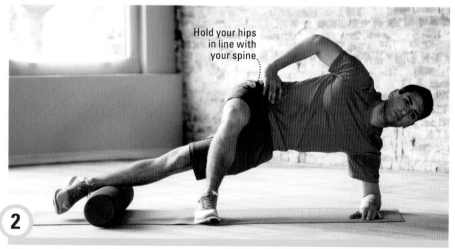

Hold your hips in line with your spine

**2**

**Lift your hips** and roll down to your ankle, pushing with your right leg.

Slightly rotate your leg in and out to release all three muscles.

Massaging the peroneals can relieve referred pain in your ankles and your feet.

**3**

**Roll up** to your knee joint. Continue to roll the length of the lower leg for 20 to 30 seconds.

**4**

**Switch the foam roller** to your lower right leg and repeat the exercise.

**CAUTION**
To avoid injury, if you feel excessive pain, then offset pressure from the roller. Shift weight to your support leg and arm, and never exceed your pain tolerance.

**MODIFICATION**

**To increase pressure,** stack both legs on top of the foam roller.

# ARCH RELEASE

This vital exercise alleviates pain from *plantar fasciitis* and restores circulation and flexibility for healthy feet. The bottom of the foot is the brain's principal input for balance and reaction time, and this exercise improves the foot's receptivity to these signals.

**TARGETED MUSCLES**

This exercise targets the *plantar fascia* in the bottom of the foot. This thick band of soft tissue connects the heel bone to the toes and supports the arch.

FRONT          BACK

**1**

**Sit in a chair** and place the massage stick on the ground beneath your right foot.

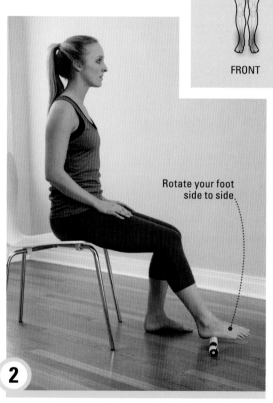

Rotate your foot side to side.

**2**

**Slide your right foot** forward and backward over the stick, from the ball to the heel of the foot, for 30 to 45 seconds. Then repeat for the left foot.

# TARGETED FOOT RELEASE

A good foot massage is relaxing and restorative, but the Targeted Foot Release can also do wonders for relieving pain caused by trigger points. If you're on your feet a lot and have tight calves or wear shoes that don't fit well, then this exercise will help.

## TARGETED MUSCLES

This release targets the seven primary muscles in the bottom of the foot, which collectively control the toes and stabilize the arch.

FRONT          BACK

Relax your toes

**1**

**Sit on the ground,** place the lacrosse ball beneath your left foot, and roll the area from the heel to the arch. If you find a painful point, massage it with circular movements for 20 to 30 seconds.

**2**

**Refocus pressure** and roll the area from the arch to the pads of the foot. Spend 20 to 30 seconds massaging painful points. Then repeat for the right foot.

## MODIFICATION

**To increase pressure,** stand upright and push your foot into the ball.

# UPPER BODY
# EXERCISES

# SPINE RESTORATION

The thoracic spine runs from the neck to the lower back, and this release restores its length and flexibility. This part of the spine is crucial for movement of the head and shoulders, so doing the exercise regularly can alleviate neck and arm problems.

## TARGETED MUSCLES

This exercise targets alignment of the thoracic spine vertebrae, from the neck to the lower back. The torso bends and twists here.

FRONT          BACK

**(1)**

**Lie with your back** on the foam roller, and plant both feet on the ground for support.

Support your head with your arms...

**(2)**

**Lift your hips** off the ground by pushing through your feet, and inhale.

## CAUTION

To prevent spinal injury, stop immediately if you experience pain in your spine. Instead, attempt the modification for less pressure.

Exhale as you pass over the midpoint of the thoracic spine

**(3)**

**Roll the length of your thoracic spine** for 20 to 30 seconds, from the shoulder blades to the bottom of the ribcage, pushing and pulling with the legs.

**(4)**

**Pick three to four points** during the movement to pause, drop your arms and hips to the ground, and exhale deeply while pushing into the roller.

## MODIFICATIONS

**To decrease pressure,** pin the roller against a wall and do slight squats to move it up and down.

**To make it harder,** reach your arms straight above your head while rolling.

# SPINE LENGTHENING

Lengthening your spine restores its natural curvature, from the base of the head to the hips. Your posture adapts to adverse lifestyle conditions, but this exercise can mitigate the discomfort. It's especially beneficial to perform before working out.

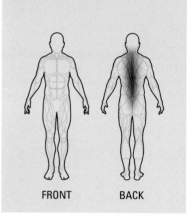

### TARGETED MUSCLES

This exercise targets the core musculature in the back. These muscles align the spine to improve total body health.

FRONT          BACK

**1**

**Lie with your back** and head on the foam roller, and plant your feet on the ground for support. Rest your arms at your sides.

### TIP

To achieve extra length in your spine, this exercise works well in combination with the Spine Restoration and Hip Flexor Release exercises.

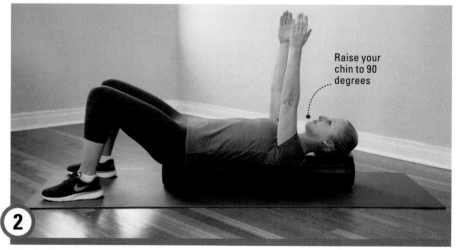

Raise your chin to 90 degrees

**2**

**Inhale deeply** through your nose and raise your arms straight up. Push your lower back into the roller.

Keep your upper back
fixed on the roller

Widen your stance
to achieve balance
and to improve
your lower back's
contact with the
foam roller.

**3**

**Exhale through your mouth** and lower your
arms straight back to lengthen your spine.

**4**

**Return your arms** to the starting position and
repeat the exercise 10 to 15 times.

**HOW IT HELPS**
Pushing your lower
back into the roller
produces a contraction
in your abdominals,
making it a great
alternative way to
strengthen the core.

**MODIFICATION**

**To increase
pressure,** bend
your knees and
rest your feet on a
chair to maximize
contact with the
roller and to ease
hip tension.

# LOWER BACK RELEASE

Foam rolling the lower back relieves the exhausted muscles that help stabilize the hips. These muscles straddle the lumbar spine and can become especially fatigued from poor posture or from running on uneven surfaces, slanted pavement, and trails.

**TARGETED MUSCLES**

This exercise targets the *quadratus lumborum,* a muscle that connects to the rib cage, pelvis, and spine as part of the body's core musculature. It helps support the spine and breathing.

FRONT          BACK

**1**

**Sit on the ground** and plant your feet in front of you. Position the foam roller behind your lower back.

**CAUTION**
To avoid damage and pain to your lumbar spine, you must only apply pressure to your muscles. Never foam roll your bones.

Use your left forearm for support

**2**

**Turn your torso** to the left, lift your hips, and apply pressure to the soft tissues on the left side of your spine, above the pelvis.

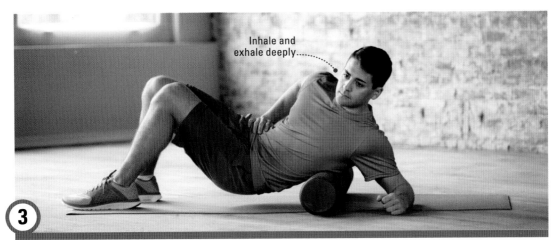

Inhale and
exhale deeply....

**3**

**Gently roll up and down** over the length of your
lower back for 20 to 30 seconds.

**4**

**Turn your torso** to the right and repeat the
exercise for your right lower back.

## TIP
To diminish leg and hip
pain, do the exercise
often and strengthen
your legs and hips.
Weak legs require the
lower back to work
especially hard
during movement.

## MODIFICATION

**To make it
easier,** use a
massage stick to
roll the soft tissue
next to your
lumbar spine.

# TARGETED LOWER BACK RELEASE

Foam rolling your lower back helps overall mobility, but targeting trigger points best controls pain in the lumbar spine. These muscles easily strain due to inactive gluteals or during loaded twisting actions, like turning and bending to pick up a child.

## TARGETED MUSCLES

This exercise targets the *quadratus lumborum*, a muscle that connects to the rib cage, pelvis, and spine as part of the body's core musculature. It helps the body bend sideways.

FRONT          BACK

**(1)**

**Stand upright** and pin the lacrosse ball between the wall and the area to the right of your spine, beneath the ribcage and above the pelvis.

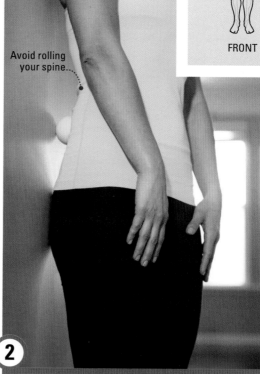

Avoid rolling your spine...

**(2)**

**Rotate to the right** to roll the ball horizontally over the muscles from the spine to your side. If you find a painful point, massage it with circular movements for 20 to 30 seconds.

Massage trigger points in your back with moderate, sustained pressure in a circular motion to reduce pain.

**3** **Bend your knees** to roll the ball vertically up your back, and spend 20 to 30 seconds massaging particularly painful points.

**4** **Rotate your body** to the left and repeat the exercise for the area to the left of your spine.

## MODIFICATION

**To increase pressure,** lie on the ground and place the lacrosse ball beneath your lower back.

### TIP
To permanently heal lower back pain, identify the cause. Trigger point release briefly helps, but weak muscles and bad habits chronically overwork the back.

# MIDDLE BACK RELEASE

Massaging the middle back balances the head and shoulder complex. If your head and arms are routinely pulled forward, then your shoulders are likely overworked at this mechanical disadvantage. Rolling the middle back reduces the tension and pain.

## TARGETED MUSCLES

This exercise targets the *trapezius*, *rhomboids*, and *serratus posterior*, muscles that straddle the spine in the middle back. They support the head and shoulder blades.

FRONT          BACK

**1**

**Lie with your back** and head on the foam roller, and plant your feet on the ground for support.

Cradle your head with your right arm.

**2**

**Rotate to the left** to focus pressure on the muscles to the left of your spine, and extend your left arm along the ground.

**3**

**Slowly roll side to side,** from your shoulder blades to your spine, for 20 to 30 seconds. Use your legs and torso to propel the movement.

**4**

**Rotate your torso** to the right and repeat the exercise for your right middle back.

## HOW IT HELPS

This exercise is a great way to ease stress. It feels like a deep tissue massage when you relax your muscles and breathe deeply.

## MODIFICATION

**To make it easier,** pin the roller against a wall with your back and lean into the roller.

# TARGETED MIDDLE BACK RELEASE

Painful trigger points often afflict the middle back. Lifting heavy objects, over-exercise, and poor posture cause deviations from your neutral spinal alignment, causing the painful points. Frequently do this easy exercise to alleviate discomfort.

## TARGETED MUSCLES

This exercise targets the superficial muscles of the middle back (those closest to the surface). They straddle the vertebrae to protect and align the spine.

FRONT          BACK

Target the muscular mounds that straddle your vertebrae

**(1)**

**Stand upright** and pin the lacrosse ball between the wall and the area to the left of the spine below the shoulder blade. Cross your left arm over your chest and lean into the ball.

Massage the trigger points in your back with moderate, sustained pressure in circular motions until the pain dissolves.

**(2)**

**Bend your knees** to roll the ball up your middle back. If you find a painful point, massage it with circular movements for 20 to 30 seconds.

**Switch the lacrosse ball** to your right middle back and repeat the exercise.

**Rotate your torso** to the right and refocus pressure closer to your spine. Spend 20 to 30 seconds massaging particularly painful points.

## HOW IT HELPS

This release alleviates referred pain in the back and lower body. Target these trigger points when you have lower back, gluteal, and leg pain.

**MODIFICATION**

**To make it easier,** place the ball in a long sock and hold it over the top of your shoulder.

# MIDDLE BACK ACTIVATION

This simple exercise restores balance to taut back muscles, which act on the shoulder complex. Inactivity in your middle back leads to an overactive upper back, causing soreness in the neck, shoulders, and arms. This is common for people who reach forward often.

## TARGETED MUSCLES

This exercise targets the *trapezius*, the diamond shaped muscle traveling from the base of the neck, out to the shoulders, and in toward the lower back. It supports the shoulder blades and arms.

FRONT          BACK

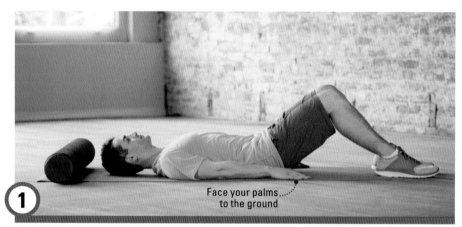

**1**

Face your palms to the ground

**Lie on your back** and plant your feet on the ground. Place the foam roller above your head.

**TIP**
To depress the shoulder blades (move them down) for an effective starting position, stretch your hands down to your feet before you begin each repetition.

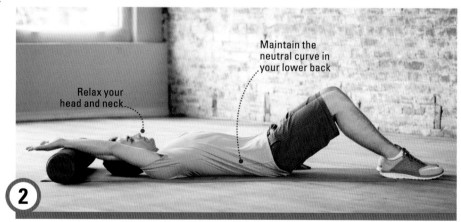

Maintain the neutral curve in your lower back

Relax your head and neck

**2**

**Arc your right arm** straight up and back. When your arm contacts the roller, press further into the roller until your middle back contracts, and hold for 3 seconds.

Feel your back
contract
between your
shoulder blades...

**3**

**Return your right arm** to the starting position,
and repeat the arcing motion with your left arm.

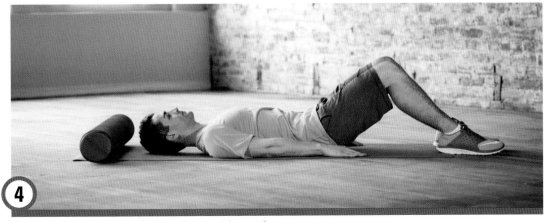

**4**

**Return your left arm** to the starting position and
repeat the exercise 10 times.

## MODIFICATIONS

**To make it
easier,** lean back
against a wall and
arc your arms to
the wall above
your head.

**To make
it harder,**
straighten your
legs to challenge
your lower back.

# TARGETED SHOULDER RELEASE

Different jobs or activities that ask you to repeatedly reach back, up, or out can overwork your shoulders. These actions cause trigger points and referred pain throughout the upper body, but doing this exercise relieves tension and improves flexibility.

**TARGETED MUSCLES**

This release targets the three distinct regions of the deltoid: anterior deltoid, lateral deltoid, and posterior deltoid. They control reaching movements.

FRONT          BACK

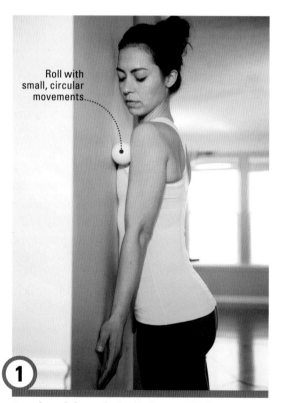

Roll with small, circular movements.

**1** **Stand upright** and pin the lacrosse ball between the wall and the front of your left shoulder. Roll the front of your shoulder for about 25 seconds.

Rotate your arm in and out while rolling.

Massage with sustained, circular movements to release the tension and trigger points in your shoulder.

**2** **Turn your body** to roll the side of your left shoulder for 20 to 30 seconds.

**Switch the lacrosse ball** to your right shoulder and repeat the exercise.

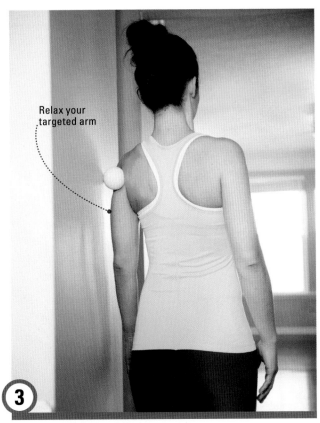

Relax your targeted arm

**Turn your body again** to roll the back of your left shoulder for 20 to 30 seconds.

### TIP
To heal incessant pain, even while at rest, look for trigger points in surrounding muscles. Trigger points in the pectorals or underarms can refer pain to the shoulders.

### MODIFICATION

**To increase pressure,** lie on the ground and place the ball beneath your shoulder.

# SHOULDER BLADE RELEASE

The shoulder blades mobilize several movements, so the many attached muscles become temperamental and overworked. If you always hold your arms in front of you—typing or on your phone—then you can benefit from this lengthening exercise.

## TARGETED MUSCLES

This exercise targets the rotator cuff muscles: the *infraspinatus*, *supraspinatus*, and *teres minor*. They stabilize the shoulder.

FRONT          BACK

Support your head with your left arm

Relax your right arm to keep tension off the rotator cuff muscles

**1**

**Lie on your back** and place the foam roller beneath your right shoulder. Plant both feet on the ground, raise your hips, and rotate your torso to the right.

Breathe deeply.

Concentrate your weight on the targeted shoulder

**2**

**TIP**

For permanently pain-free shoulders, determine the cause and adjust bad habits. For example, pull the keyboard closer to you when typing.

**Roll back and forth** over your right shoulder blade for 20 to 30 seconds, pushing and pulling with your legs. Then rotate your torso to the left and repeat the exercise for your left shoulder.

# FRONT SHOULDER RELEASE

Releasing the front of your shoulder restores healthy range-of-motion in your arm and alleviates pain in surrounding areas. Overhead athletes like baseball and volleyball players especially benefit from improved flexibility by doing this exercise.

## TARGETED MUSCLES

This exercise targets the anterior deltoid in the front of the shoulder. This part of the deltoid lifts the arm away from the body.

FRONT          BACK

Face your right palm down and relax the hand

**1**

**Lie on your stomach** and extend your right arm to 90 degrees. Place the foam roller beneath the front of your right shoulder.

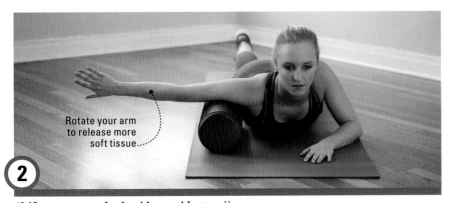

Rotate your arm to release more soft tissue

**2**

**Shift your upper body side-to-side** to roll the width of your right shoulder for 20 to 30 seconds. Then switch the foam roller to your left shoulder and repeat the exercise.

## MODIFICATION

**To decrease pressure,** extend your arm and pin the foam roller between the wall and your front shoulder.

# SHOULDER BLADE MOBILIZATION

For more effective pushing and pulling and a healthier rotator cuff, use this exercise to develop shoulder blade stability and mobility. A stable shoulder blade produces efficient protraction and retraction and helps alleviate shoulder, back, and neck pain.

## TARGETED MUSCLES

This exercise targets the *serratus anterior* (beneath the shoulder blade) and the rhomboid (between the shoulder blade and spine). They stabilize the shoulder blades.

FRONT          BACK

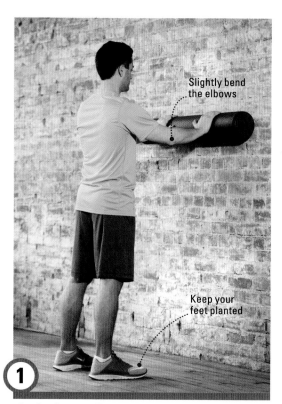

Slightly bend the elbows

Keep your feet planted

Keep your head raised

**1**

**Pin the foam roller to the wall** with the hands at shoulder height. Extend your arms. Lean forward.

**2**

**Retract, or draw your shoulder blades together,** so that you move slightly toward the wall.

To improve the stability of your shoulder joints, keep the hands fixed and upright on the roller.

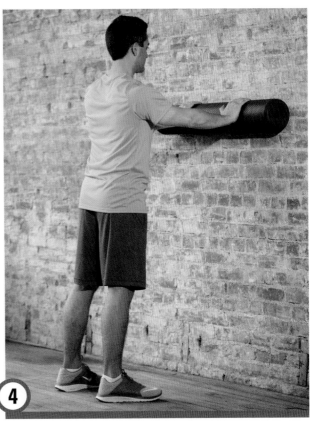

**3** **Protract, or pull your shoulder blades apart,** so that you move away from the wall. At the same time, rotate the elbows in and hold for 2 seconds.

**4** **Return to the starting position** and repeat the exercise 10 times.

## MODIFICATIONS

**To increase pressure,** plant your feet farther from the wall.

**To make it harder,** do the exercise from a push-up position on the ground.

# CHEST RELEASE

Tension in one muscle group can refer pain to the opposing muscle group, so a tight chest can cause trigger points in the upper back and shoulders. Use this exercise to restore circulation and reduce referred pain in your upper body.

## TARGETED MUSCLES

This exercise targets the *pectoralis major* and *pectoralis minor* of the chest. These muscles pull the arms forward.

FRONT　　BACK

**(1)** Lie on your stomach and extend your left arm along the ground. Place the foam roller beneath your left underarm.

**TIP**
To make the exercise easier, you can use your opposite hand to turn the roller and facilitate the movement.

**(2)** Roll up to your upper arm, pulling with your feet, and rotate your palm up.

Completely relax your arm

**3**

**Roll down** to your sternum and rotate your palm down. Continue to roll the shoulder-chest junction for 20 to 30 seconds.

**4**

**Switch the foam roller** to your right underarm and repeat the exercise.

**HOW IT HELPS**
Massaging the chest reduces stiffness and pain if you spend excessive time holding your arms forward for activities like typing and driving.

**MODIFICATION**

**To make it easier,** pin the roller to a wall with your chest.

# TARGETED CHEST RELEASE

If you have a desk job, your chest may be laden with trigger points. Prolonged sitting pulls your shoulders forward, which shortens the chest muscles and causes pain. Using a ball to release the muscles will alleviate soreness and improve flexibility.

## TARGETED MUSCLES

This release targets the *pectoralis major* and *pectoralis minor* in the chest. These pull and rotate the arms toward the body's center.

FRONT          BACK

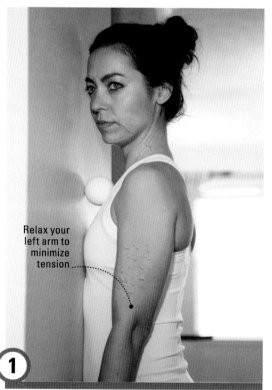

Relax your left arm to minimize tension

**1**

**Stand upright** and pin the lacrosse ball between the wall and your left pectoral region, beneath the collarbone. Lean into the ball.

The ball will move only slightly with this shift

**2**

Sustained massage and moderate pressure to this area make the chest feel looser and breathing easier.

**Shift side-to-side** to roll the ball across your upper chest. If you find a painful point, massage it with circular movements for 20 to 30 seconds.

**Switch the lacrosse ball** to your right side and repeat the exercise.

**Move the ball** to your lower chest and raise your left arm. Shift side-to-side to roll the ball across your lower chest, and spend 20 to 30 seconds massaging particularly painful points.

**HOW IT HELPS**

This release soothes upper body pain if you carry a large bag or backpack. But for a permanent solution, you must actively change your habits.

**MODIFICATION**

**To access other trigger points,** lie on the ground, place the ball beneath your chest, and slowly arc your arm.

# LATS RELEASE

To alleviate tension in and around your shoulders, the Lats Release elongates the muscles and restores overhead function. If you lift overhead or hold your arms at your side for extended periods, you'll benefit from massaging this area of your back.

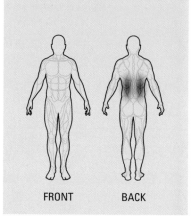

**TARGETED MUSCLES**

This exercise targets the *latissimus dorsi* (lat), the broadest muscle in the back. It controls the shoulder and pulling movements.

FRONT          BACK

Slightly rotate your torso backward to place pressure on the soft tissue

**1**

**Lie on your right side,** place the foam roller beneath your right underarm, and plant your left foot on the ground for support.

Relax your right arm

**2**

**Lift your hips** and roll down to the shoulder blade, pushing with your left arm and leg.

Pressure to the muscle at the bottom of your ribcage restores balance to the muscles that pull on your shoulders.

**3**

**Rotate your torso back** and roll to the bottom of your ribcage. Continue to roll the length of your right lat for 20 to 30 seconds.

**4**

**Switch the foam roller** to your left side and repeat the exercise.

**TIP**

To follow the lat muscle, which wraps around your back and side, rotate your ribcage forward and backward as you roll.

**MODIFICATION**

**To make it easier,** extend your arm along a wall, pin the roller to the wall with your side, and bend your knees to move the roller.

# UNDERARM RELEASE

The small movement of this exercise targets the area where the arms join the ribcage. If you keep your arms close to your sides a lot, these muscles can become taut and painful, but foam rolling the underarm can restore length and circulation.

## TARGETED MUSCLES

This exercise targets the *infraspinatus, teres major,* and *teres minor,* the muscles in the underarms. They help stabilize the humerus (upper-arm bone).

FRONT        BACK

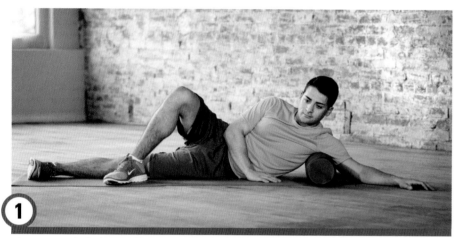

**①**

**Lie on your left side,** place the foam roller beneath your left underarm, and plant your right foot on the ground for support.

Use your right arm to facilitate the rotation of your torso or the movement of the foam roller.

Relax your extended arm

**②**

**Rotate your torso forward** and roll up to your upper arm, pulling with your right foot.

**(3)**

**Rotate your torso and left arm back** and roll
to the bottom of your underarm. Continue to roll
the length of the underarm for 20 to 30 seconds.

**(4)**

**Switch the foam roller** to your right underarm
and repeat the exercise.

## HOW IT HELPS

This release restores balance in the shoulder complex by increasing flexibility in certain muscles and decreasing tension in opposing muscles.

## MODIFICATION

**To make it easier,**
extend your arm along
a wall and pin the
roller to the wall with
your underarm.

# BICEPS RELEASE

If you hold heavy objects with a flexed elbow, you may develop pain in the biceps. Massage this muscle group to improve circulation and alleviate tension. You can trace many disorders of the hand, wrist, elbow, and shoulder to chronically tight biceps.

## TARGETED MUSCLES

This exercise targets the biceps muscle group, located in the inner, upper arm. These muscles help flex the elbow, rotate the forearm, and stabilize the shoulder blade.

FRONT          BACK

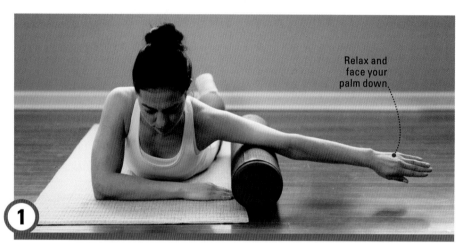

Relax and face your palm down.

**1**

**Lie on your stomach** and extend your left arm to 90 degrees. Place the foam roller beneath your left biceps.

**2**

**Shift your upper body side-to-side** to roll the length of your left biceps for 20 to 30 seconds, from your shoulder to your elbow.

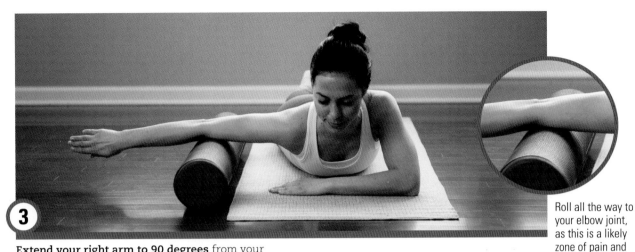

**3**

Extend your right arm to 90 degrees from your body and switch the roller to your right biceps.

Roll all the way to your elbow joint, as this is a likely zone of pain and trigger points.

**4**

Shift your upper body side-to-side to roll the length of your right biceps for 20 to 30 seconds, from your shoulder to your elbow.

**TIP**
To restore balance to your muscle groups, also do the Chest Release exercise and any shoulder release exercises to improve flexibility of the arms and upper body.

**MODIFICATION**

**To make it easier,** pin the foam roller to the wall with your biceps.

# TRICEPS RELEASE

For elbow and shoulder pain, the Triceps Release can relieve referred pain. Repetitively extending the elbow joint, whether at your job or while playing a sport, can burden your triceps with sensitive trigger points that the foam roller can release.

## TARGETED MUSCLES

This exercise targets the triceps muscle group, located in the back of the upper arm. They extend the elbow and stabilize the shoulder.

FRONT          BACK

Rotate your arm up to access the triceps

**1**

**Lie on your left side,** place the foam roller beneath your left arm, and plant your right foot on the ground for support.

**2**

**Roll down** to your elbow joint, pushing with your right arm and right leg.

It's important to rotate your arm as much as possible to access the triceps in the back.

Relax the hand of your targeted arm

**3** **Roll up** to your underarm. Continue to roll the length of the triceps for 20 to 30 seconds.

**4** **Switch the foam roller** to your right triceps and repeat the exercise.

## HOW IT HELPS
This exercise alleviates pain in the elbow joint, common in tennis players and golfers who repetitively and forcefully extend the elbow.

# FOREARM WALL SLIDE

This wall slide establishes shoulder mobility in an overhead position. If you load your shoulder joint for activities like painting a wall or putting luggage in an overhead compartment, then mobilize your shoulders so you're not vulnerable to injury.

**TARGETED MUSCLES**

This exercise targets the *serratus anterior* (located along the sides of the ribcage). This muscle rotates the shoulder blades upward.

FRONT          BACK

Apply pressure into the wall with your arms to produce the contraction, but don't lean forward.

**1** **Stand about 1 foot (31cm) from the wall** with your feet shoulder-width apart. Pin the foam roller to the wall with the sides of your hands.

**2** **Apply pressure into the roller** through your hands. Slowly glide your forearms up over the roller without raising your shoulders.

**4**

**Return your arms** to the starting position and repeat the exercise 10 times.

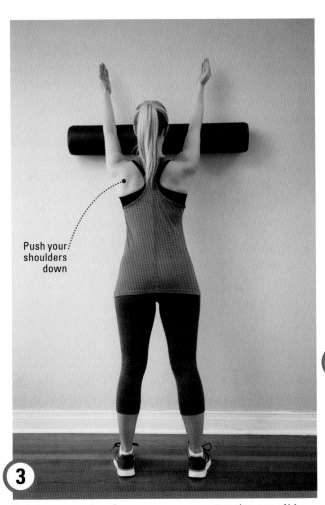

Push your shoulders down

**3**

**Rotate your palms in** as you move up. Continue to glide up until you fully extend your arms.

**TIP**

To target the correct muscle, begin by drawing your shoulder blades together. The key is to slide as high as you can without lifting the shoulders.

# NECK RELEASE

Rolling the back of the neck helps if you habitually look down. A chronic forward head position overworks the muscles that insert into the base of the skull, but rolling the back of the neck helps alleviate the tension and even reduce headaches.

**TARGETED MUSCLES**

This exercise targets the upper *trapezius*, the *levator scapulae*, and the deep neck extensors in the back of the neck. These influence the position of the head.

FRONT          BACK

**(1)**

Stand **comfortably** and hold the massage stick against the right side of your neck.

Firmly hold the stick and push forward to produce moderate pressure.

Place moderate pressure on the soft tissue, not the spine.

**(2)**

Turn **your head** to the right and roll up the right side of your neck to your ear.

**3**

**Roll down** the right side of your neck to your shoulders. Continue to roll the length of the right side of your neck for 20 to 30 seconds.

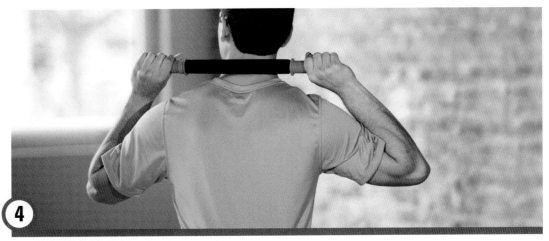

**4**

**Turn your head** to the left and repeat the exercise for the left side of your neck.

## HOW IT HELPS

This exercise reduces tension from "text neck" if you habitually look down at a phone. Try using your eye muscles instead of the neck to look down.

## MODIFICATION

**To make it easier,** place a foam roller beneath your neck and slowly turn your head from side to side.

# FINGER FLEXOR RELEASE

You use the network of hand and finger flexors any time you carry a bag, type, or shake hands. They pull your hand and fingers inward, but over- and underuse can cause tightness. Use this exercise to reduce the pain and tension.

## TARGETED MUSCLES

This exercise targets the hand and finger flexors, which originate near the inside of the elbow. They bend the hand inward and clench the fingers and thumb.

FRONT          BACK

**1**

**Pin the lacrosse ball** between the wall and the inside of your right forearm, flatten your palm against the wall, and lean into the ball.

**2**

**Move the right forearm up** to roll the ball over the flexors. If you find a painful point, massage it with circular movements for 20 to 30 seconds. Then repeat the exercise for your left arm.

# FINGER EXTENSOR RELEASE

When you straighten, lift, stretch, or point your fingers, you use your hand and finger extensors. These are prone to overuse and injury, especially if you type on a misplaced keyboard with your wrists lower than the keys. Perform this exercise to relieve pain.

## TARGETED MUSCLES

This exercise targets the hand and finger extensors, which originate near the outside of the elbow. They bend the hand backward and lift the fingers and thumb.

FRONT          BACK

Relax your fingers to better penetrate trigger points.

**1** **Pin the lacrosse ball** between the wall and the outside of your right forearm. Lean into the ball.

**2** **Bend your knees** to roll the ball over the extensors. If you find a painful point, massage it with circular movements for 20 to 30 seconds. Then repeat the exercise for your left arm.

# TARGETED PALM RELEASE

You use your hands for almost every activity during the day, from signing a check to grasping a bag. You can easily overwork the muscles in your palm, so do this exercise frequently as a simple cure for trigger points and tension in your hands.

## TARGETED MUSCLES

This release targets the four largest muscles in the hand. They control movements of the thumb.

FRONT          BACK

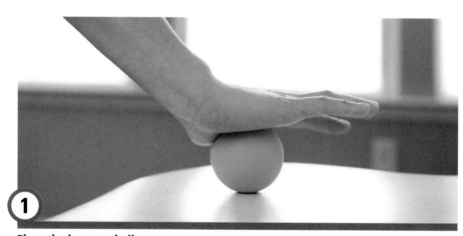

**1**

**Place the lacrosse ball** on an elevated surface and rest your right palm on the ball.

**HOW IT HELPS**
Rolling the hands stimulates the nerves in your skin to send proprioceptive information to your body and improve your coordination.

Massage with sustained, circular movements.

**2**

**Press your right hand** into the ball with the left hand and massage the area between your palm and thumb for 20 to 30 seconds.

**3**

**Glide the rest of your palm** over the ball. If you find a particularly painful point, massage it with circular movements for 20 to 30 seconds.

**4**

**Switch the lacrosse ball** to your left hand and repeat the exercise.

# PAIN RELIEF
# PROGRAMS

# UPPER BACK

Reaching to a keyboard or looking down at a cell phone strains the upper back, as certain muscles become overworked and others underworked. To reduce pain, do these exercises to improve your back's strength and flexibility.

## WHAT YOU NEED

Foam roller

Chair

Yoga mat

## WHAT TO DO

○ Do the exercises in order.
○ Spend 30 to 45 seconds on each exercise.
○ Breathe deeply and relax your muscles.
○ Devote extra time to releasing more painful upper body muscles.

| | EXERCISE | TOOL | PAGE |
|---|---|---|---|
| 1 | CHEST RELEASE | | P118 |
| 2 | FRONT SHOULDER RELEASE | | P115 |
| 3 | SPINE RESTORATION | | P98 |
| 4 | SPINE LENGTHENING | | P100 |
| 5 | SITTING RIBCAGE ROTATION | | P34 |
| 6 | MIDDLE BACK ACTIVATION | | P110 |
| 7 | PLANK PROGRESSIONS | | P24 |

SPINE LENGTHENING

**TIP**
For lasting upper back relief, actively correct your posture. Lengthen the torso and retract your shoulder blades.

# LOWER BACK

When your hips are immobile or tight, the lower back compensates, causing trigger points and poor alignment. Complete this program to activate your hip muscles, massage the related muscles, and relieve lower back discomfort.

## WHAT YOU NEED

- Foam roller
- Lacrosse ball
- Yoga mat

## WHAT TO DO

○ Do the exercises in order.

○ Spend 30 to 45 seconds on each exercise.

○ Monitor your pain level and adjust pressure accordingly.

○ Focus pressure on your soft tissue, and avoid rolling bones.

| | EXERCISE | TOOL | PAGE |
|---|---|---|---|
| 1 | HIP FLEXOR RELEASE | | P50 |
| 2 | HAMSTRINGS RELEASE | | P72 |
| 3 | SPINE RESTORATION | | P98 |
| 4 | LOWER BACK RELEASE | | P102 |
| 5 | TARGETED LOWER BACK RELEASE | | P104 |
| 6 | SPINE LENGTHENING | | P100 |
| 7 | BIRD DOG REACH | | P30 |

LOWER BACK RELEASE

# SHOULDER AND NECK

Joints and soft tissues in your neck and shoulders easily strain if you frequently use your arms to reach overhead and forward, if you have poor posture, or if you rarely use your upper body during the day. Do these exercises to subdue the pain.

## WHAT YOU NEED

- Massage stick
- Foam roller
- Yoga mat

## WHAT TO DO

- Do the exercises in order.
- Spend 30 to 45 seconds on each exercise.
- Monitor your pain level and adjust pressure accordingly.
- Relax your neck and arm muscles so you're more receptive to release.

| | EXERCISE | TOOL | PAGE |
|---|---|---|---|
| 1 | NECK RELEASE | | P132 |
| 2 | SHOULDER BLADE RELEASE | | P114 |
| 3 | SPINE LENGTHENING | | P100 |
| 4 | CHEST RELEASE | | P118 |
| 5 | MIDDLE BACK RELEASE | | P106 |

SHOULDER BLADE RELEASE ▶

# TARGETED SHOULDER AND NECK

If you have sharp pain or tightness in the shoulders or neck, you likely have many over- and underused muscles that refer pain through the area. Complete this program to relieve the trigger points and secure pain-free posture.

## WHAT YOU NEED

- ◯ Lacrosse ball
- ▱ Foam roller
- ◇ Yoga mat

## WHAT TO DO

- Do the exercises in order.
- Spend 30 to 45 seconds on each exercise.
- Breathe deeply and relax your muscles.
- Find the trigger points that refer pain through your shoulders and neck.

| | EXERCISE | TOOL | PAGE |
|---|---|---|---|
| 1 | TARGETED MIDDLE BACK RELEASE | ◯ | P108 |
| 2 | TARGETED SHOULDER RELEASE | ◯ | P112 |
| 3 | SHOULDER BLADE RELEASE | ▱ | P114 |
| 4 | TARGETED CHEST RELEASE | ◯ | P120 |
| 5 | UNDERARM RELEASE | ▱ | P124 |

# HIPS

Several muscles originate and insert around the pelvis, making your hips prone to tightness and pain. Use this program to improve flexibility and muscle health in the overworked or underworked hips and related muscles.

## WHAT YOU NEED

- Foam roller
- Lacrosse ball
- Yoga mat

## WHAT TO DO

- Do the exercises in order.
- Spend 30 to 45 seconds on each exercise.
- Breathe deeply and relax your muscles.
- Repeat the exercises that target your most tense muscles.

| # | EXERCISE | TOOL | PAGE |
|---|----------|------|------|
| 1 | HIP FLEXOR RELEASE | Foam roller | P50 |
| 2 | GLUTEAL GROUP RELEASE | Foam roller | P58 |
| 3 | QUADRICEPS RELEASE | Foam roller | P66 |
| 4 | OUTER THIGH AND HIP RELEASE | Foam roller | P70 |
| 5 | INNER THIGH RELEASE | Foam roller | P76 |
| 6 | HAMSTRINGS RELEASE | Foam roller | P72 |
| 7 | TARGETED HIP ROTATOR RELEASE | Lacrosse ball | P52 |

OUTER THIGH AND HIP RELEASE ▶

**HOW IT HELPS**
Massaging the hips and upper legs can soothe debilitating hip pain while sitting, standing, walking, and running.

# UPPER LEGS

From athletics to frequent sitting, many activities cause knee and hip pain. Disorders of the upper legs often originate from weak or misused muscles, but doing these exercises relieves pain and strengthens your upper legs.

## WHAT YOU NEED

- Foam roller
- Lacrosse ball
- Chair
- Yoga mat

## WHAT TO DO

- Do the exercises in order.
- Spend 30 to 45 seconds on each exercise.
- Monitor your pain level and adjust pressure accordingly.
- Maximize soft tissue release by rotating your legs during the exercises.

| | EXERCISE | TOOL | PAGE |
|---|---|---|---|
| 1 | QUADRICEPS RELEASE | | P66 |
| 2 | OUTER THIGH AND HIP RELEASE | | P70 |
| 3 | TARGETED HIP FLEXOR RELEASE | | P51 |
| 4 | TARGETED HAMSTRINGS RELEASE | | P74 |
| 5 | TARGETED INNER THIGH RELEASE | | P78 |
| 6 | CLAMSHELL HIP ROTATION | | P56 |
| 7 | HIP ROTATOR RAISE | | P54 |

QUADRICEPS RELEASE ▶

# LOWER LEGS

You don't have to be an avid runner to develop lower leg pain—sometimes even pressing the gas and brake pedals repeatedly will cause pain. Your lower legs are often overworked, so do these exercises to alleviate discomfort.

## WHAT YOU NEED

Foam roller

Massage stick

Chair

Yoga mat

## WHAT TO DO

- Do the exercises in order.
- Spend 30 to 45 seconds on each exercise.
- Breathe deeply and relax your muscles.
- Keep your feet and ankles loose so that your legs are receptive to release.

| EXERCISE | TOOL | PAGE |
|---|---|---|
| 1 CALF MASSAGE | | P86 |
| 2 KNEE RELEASE | | P80 |
| 3 SHIN RELEASE | | P82 |
| 4 ANKLE RELEASE | | P92 |
| 5 ARCH RELEASE | | P94 |

CALF MASSAGE

# HAND AND FOREARM

As many desk workers, pianists, or tennis players could attest, pain in the forearms and hands can be debilitating in day-to-day activities like opening a jar or brushing your teeth. Follow this program to keep pain in your arms at bay.

## WHAT YOU NEED

- Lacrosse ball
- Foam roller
- Yoga mat

## WHAT TO DO

- Do the exercises in order.
- Spend 30 to 45 seconds on each exercise.
- Monitor your pain level and adjust pressure accordingly.
- Relax your hands and wrists.

| | EXERCISE | TOOL | PAGE |
|---|---|---|---|
| 1 | FINGER FLEXOR RELEASE | ◯ | P134 |
| 2 | FINGER EXTENSOR RELEASE | ◯ | P135 |
| 3 | TARGETED PALM RELEASE | ◯ | P136 |
| 4 | TRICEPS RELEASE | ▭ | P128 |
| 5 | BICEPS RELEASE | ▭ | P126 |
| 6 | CHEST RELEASE | ▭ | P118 |

# FEET

When you're always wearing socks and shoes, your feet easily become desensitized and painful while diminishing your body awareness. Complete these exercises to prevent or alleviate foot pain and improve your balance.

## WHAT YOU NEED

- Massage stick
- Lacrosse ball
- Foam roller
- Half roller
- Chair
- Yoga mat

## WHAT TO DO

- Do the exercises in order.
- Spend 30 to 45 seconds on each exercise.
- Breathe deeply and relax your targeted foot.
- Remove your socks and shoes.

| | EXERCISE | TOOL | PAGE |
|---|---|---|---|
| 1 | ARCH RELEASE | | P94 |
| 2 | TARGETED CALF RELEASE | | P88 |
| 3 | ANKLE RELEASE | | P92 |
| 4 | TARGETED FOOT RELEASE | | P95 |
| 5 | SPIRAL CALF RAISE | | P90 |

### HOW IT HELPS

Massaging your soles sharpens sensory input from thousands of nerve endings, even when you're wearing shoes.

TARGETED PALM RELEASE

# LIFESTYLE
# PROGRAMS

# TOO MUCH SITTING

Sitting too much is detrimental, as it deteriorates your posture and imbalances your muscles. The result is a myriad of pains and stiff joints throughout your body. Use this program to counteract the tension and re-establish mobility.

## WHAT YOU NEED

- Foam roller
- Half roller
- Yoga mat

## WHAT TO DO

- Do the exercises in order.
- Spend 30 to 45 seconds on each exercise.
- Breathe deeply and relax your muscles.
- Use a textured roller for muscles that are especially inhibited.

| | EXERCISE | TOOL | PAGE |
|---|---|---|---|
| 1 | HIP FLEXOR RELEASE | | P50 |
| 2 | QUADRICEPS RELEASE | | P66 |
| 3 | HAMSTRINGS RELEASE | | P72 |
| 4 | SPINE RESTORATION | | P98 |
| 5 | SPINE LENGTHENING | | P100 |
| 6 | GLUTEAL BRIDGE | | P62 |
| 7 | FOREARM WALL SLIDE | | P130 |
| 8 | OVERHEAD SQUAT | | P44 |
| 9 | PLANK PROGRESSIONS | | P24 |

HIP FLEXOR RELEASE

**TIP**
To limit your time seated at work, raise your desk or your computer so you're able to stand.

# TOO MUCH STANDING

Professions that require too much standing, like restaurant or retail jobs, can freeze your muscles and joints into one position and make them stiff and imbalanced. Do this program to restore functional movement and limit trigger points.

## WHAT YOU NEED

- Foam roller
- Massage stick
- Chair
- Yoga mat

## WHAT TO DO

- Do the exercises in order.
- Spend 30 to 45 seconds on each exercise.
- Monitor your pain level and adjust pressure accordingly.
- Remove your shoes for improved body awareness.

| | EXERCISE | TOOL | PAGE |
|---|---|---|---|
| 1 | GLUTEAL GROUP RELEASE | | P58 |
| 2 | QUADRICEPS RELEASE | | P66 |
| 3 | HAMSTRINGS RELEASE | | P72 |
| 4 | CALF MASSAGE | | P86 |
| 5 | ARCH RELEASE | | P94 |
| 6 | STRAIGHT-LEG RAISE | | P40 |
| 7 | ROLLER WALKOUT | | P28 |
| 8 | HALF-KNEELING CORE ROTATION | | P36 |
| 9 | STRAIGHT-LEG GLUTEAL BRIDGE | | P64 |

GLUTEAL GROUP RELEASE

**TIP**
For healthier feet, strengthen the muscles by spending more time barefoot before resorting to inserts.

# ACTIVE LIFESTYLE

Walking a dog, gardening in the backyard, or taking care of children require mobility in several key areas and core stability to protect your spine. Do this program regularly to support the dynamic movements of your active lifestyle.

## WHAT YOU NEED

- Foam roller
- Chair
- Yoga mat

## WHAT TO DO

- Do the exercises in order.
- Spend 30 to 45 seconds on each exercise.
- Breathe deeply and relax your muscles.
- Modify the exercise or go to the next one if it's too difficult to maintain perfect posture.

| | EXERCISE | TOOL | PAGE |
|---|---|---|---|
| 1 | SPINE RESTORATION | | P98 |
| 2 | LATS RELEASE | | P122 |
| 3 | BIRD DOG REACH | | P30 |
| 4 | SPINE LENGTHENING | | P100 |
| 5 | FOREARM WALL SLIDE | | P130 |
| 6 | ADDUCTOR CHAIR SQUAT | | P48 |
| 7 | PLANK PROGRESSIONS | | P24 |
| 8 | SITTING RIBCAGE ROTATION | | P34 |

ADDUCTOR CHAIR SQUAT ▶

# DAILY CONDITIONING

Massaging your muscles and doing rotational exercises on a daily basis will make your body feel more awake and capable during day-to-day movements. Follow this easy-to-perform program to prime your body for a productive day.

## WHAT YOU NEED

○ Lacrosse ball
▭ Full roller
▱ Yoga mat

## WHAT TO DO

○ Do the exercises in order.
○ Spend 30 to 45 seconds on each exercise.
○ Monitor your pain level and adjust pressure accordingly.
○ Breathe deeply to relax your body.

| EXERCISE | TOOL | PAGE |
|---|---|---|
| 1 TARGETED FOOT RELEASE | ○ | P95 |
| 2 OUTER THIGH AND HIP RELEASE | ▭ | P70 |
| 3 INNER THIGH RELEASE | ▭ | P76 |
| 4 SPINE RESTORATION | ▭ | P98 |
| 5 SIDE-LYING RIBCAGE ROTATION | ▭ | P38 |
| 6 HIP SWIVEL | ▭ | P32 |

# OVERHEAD REACHING RELIEF

Cleaning a window, stocking a shelf, and writing on a blackboard easily overworks and strains your arms and shoulders. For people required to reach overhead often, complete these exercises to loosen the muscles and prevent injury.

## WHAT YOU NEED

- Foam roller
- Lacrosse ball
- Massage stick
- Yoga mat

## WHAT TO DO

- Do the exercises in order.
- Spend 30 to 45 seconds on each exercise.
- Breathe deeply and relax your muscles.
- Monitor the pain level in your shoulders, and adjust pressure accordingly.

| | EXERCISE | TOOL | PAGE |
|---|---|---|---|
| 1 | SPINE RESTORATION | | P98 |
| 2 | TARGETED SHOULDER RELEASE | | P112 |
| 3 | LATS RELEASE | | P122 |
| 4 | NECK RELEASE | | P132 |
| 5 | TARGETED MIDDLE BACK RELEASE | | P108 |
| 6 | SHOULDER BLADE MOBILIZATION | | P116 |
| 7 | SPINE LENGTHENING | | P100 |

OUTER THIGH AND HIP RELEASE

# POSTURE RESTORATION

Anything from tightly fitted clothing to bucket seats in a car can contribute to poor posture. Even athletics like rowing and cycling are detrimental to spine health. Perform these exercises regularly to restore your alignment.

## WHAT YOU NEED

- Foam roller
- Half roller
- Yoga mat

## WHAT TO DO

- Do the exercises in order.
- Spend 30 to 45 seconds on each exercise.
- Monitor your pain level and adjust pressure accordingly.
- Modify any exercise that becomes too easy, or increase your repetitions.

| | EXERCISE | TOOL | PAGE |
|---|---|---|---|
| 1 | SPINE RESTORATION | | P98 |
| 2 | SPINE LENGTHENING | | P100 |
| 3 | LATS RELEASE | | P122 |
| 4 | FOREARM WALL SLIDE | | P130 |
| 5 | QUADRICEPS RELEASE | | P66 |
| 6 | GLUTEAL BRIDGE | | P62 |
| 7 | ROLLER ROLLOUT | | P26 |
| 8 | STRAIGHT-LEG RAISE | | P40 |
| 9 | OVERHEAD SQUAT | | P44 |

LATS RELEASE ▶

# STRESS RELIEF

Whatever the stressors in your life, they often translate into muscle tension. The exercises in this program will release the areas where you may tend to carry the most pressure so your body can feel lighter, looser, and pain-free.

## WHAT YOU NEED

- Lacrosse ball
- Massage stick
- Foam roller
- Yoga mat

## WHAT TO DO

- Do the exercises in order.
- Spend 30 to 45 seconds on each exercise.
- Breathe deeply and relax your muscles.
- Set aside 10 minutes for the exercises in a quiet, distraction-free environment.

| | EXERCISE | TOOL | PAGE |
|---|---|---|---|
| 1 | TARGETED PALM RELEASE | | P136 |
| 2 | NECK RELEASE | | P132 |
| 3 | TARGETED SHOULDER RELEASE | | P112 |
| 4 | TARGETED MIDDLE BACK RELEASE | | P108 |
| 5 | TARGETED HIP ROTATOR RELEASE | | P52 |
| 6 | TARGETED FOOT RELEASE | | P95 |
| 7 | SPINE LENGTHENING | | P100 |

# LIMITED MOBILITY

Joints conform to the positions in which you most frequently hold them, so if you're in one position for extended periods, your joints can lose mobility. Perform these exercises to counteract the most commonly stiff joints in your body.

## WHAT YOU NEED

Foam roller

Chair

Yoga mat

## WHAT TO DO

○ Do the exercises in order.

○ Spend 30 to 45 seconds on each exercise.

○ Monitor your pain level and adjust pressure accordingly.

○ Modify the exercise if it's difficult to maintain good posture.

| | EXERCISE | TOOL | PAGE |
|---|---|---|---|
| 1 | HIP FLEXOR RELEASE | | P50 |
| 2 | QUADRICEPS RELEASE | | P66 |
| 3 | SPINE RESTORATION | | P98 |
| 4 | FOREARM WALL SLIDE | | P130 |
| 5 | ROLLER WALKOUT | | P28 |
| 6 | SITTING RIBCAGE ROTATION | | P34 |
| 7 | HALF-KNEELING CORE ROTATION | | P36 |

**HOW IT HELPS**

Foam rolling the muscle around your joints breaks up adhesions from injury and improves flexibility.

# FULL BODY RELAXATION

This program is perfect for the end of the day when you need to relax. It's only five exercises, so spend extra time on the ones that feel best. With slow, deep breathing, you'll feel the tension melt away after completing the exercise.

## WHAT YOU NEED

- Lacrosse ball
- Foam roller
- Massage stick
- Yoga mat

## WHAT TO DO

- Do the exercises in order.
- Spend 30 to 45 seconds on each exercise.
- Breathe deeply and relax your muscles.
- Remove distractions from the area and allow your muscles to melt over the tools.

| | EXERCISE | TOOL | PAGE |
|---|---|---|---|
| 1 | TARGETED LOWER BACK RELEASE | | P104 |
| 2 | MIDDLE BACK RELEASE | | P106 |
| 3 | SPINE RESTORATION | | P98 |
| 4 | SPINE LENGTHENING | | P100 |
| 5 | NECK RELEASE | | P132 |

### HOW IT HELPS

When you ease muscle tension, your heart rate slows, your breathing relaxes, and your body begins to heal.

TARGETED LOWER BACK RELEASE

# WEEKEND WARRIOR

If you're a desk worker by weekday but a warrior by weekend, do this program to complement your ambitious fitness endeavors. This well-rounded routine awakens the muscles before a workout. Or even do it briskly as your main workout.

## WHAT YOU NEED

- ◯ Lacrosse ball
- ⬭ Foam roller
- ◇ Yoga mat

## WHAT TO DO

- Do the exercises in order.
- Spend 30 to 45 seconds on each exercise.
- Breathe deeply and relax your muscles.
- Remove your shoes for the first exercise to improve balance for the remaining ones.

| | EXERCISE | TOOL | PAGE |
|---|---|---|---|
| 1 | TARGETED FOOT RELEASE | ◯ | P95 |
| 2 | SPINE RESTORATION | ⬭ | P98 |
| 3 | HIP FLEXOR RELEASE | ⬭ | P50 |
| 4 | GLUTEAL BRIDGE | ⬭ | P62 |
| 5 | CLAMSHELL HIP ROTATION | ⬭ | P56 |
| 6 | STRAIGHT-LEG RAISE | ⬭ | P40 |
| 7 | BIRD DOG REACH | ⬭ | P30 |
| 8 | HIP SWIVEL | ⬭ | P32 |
| 9 | ADDUCTOR CHAIR SQUAT | ⬭ | P48 |

TARGETED FOOT RELEASE

# LIFETIME MOBILITY

With age, mobility can gradually diminish. Proactively foam roll your muscles to lessen your chances of encountering mobility-related injuries. These exercises will keep your muscles flexible and your body awareness high.

## WHAT YOU NEED

Foam roller

Lacrosse ball

Yoga mat

## WHAT TO DO

- Do the exercises in order.
- Spend 30 to 45 seconds on each exercise.
- Monitor your pain level and adjust pressure accordingly.
- Perform the exercise against a wall or in a chair when it's difficult to get into position.

| | EXERCISE | TOOL | PAGE |
|---|---|---|---|
| 1 | CHEST RELEASE | | P118 |
| 2 | MIDDLE BACK ACTIVATION | | P110 |
| 3 | TARGETED HIP FLEXOR RELEASE | | P51 |
| 4 | TARGETED SHIN RELEASE | | P84 |
| 5 | BIRD DOG REACH | | P30 |
| 6 | TARGETED FOOT RELEASE | | P95 |

## TIP

For healthy aging and strength, it's important to stay active. Exercise significantly reduces mobility risk.

# PAIN MANAGEMENT

The stresses of your life can sometimes be enough to produce trigger points that refer pain through your whole body. If you feel an overall ache in your joints and muscles, do this program to tackle common areas of tightness.

## WHAT YOU NEED

- Lacrosse ball
- Massage stick
- Chair
- Yoga mat

## WHAT TO DO

- Do the exercises in order.
- Spend 30 to 45 seconds on each exercise.
- Breathe deeply and relax your muscles.
- Increase or decrease pressure to maintain a productive level of discomfort.

| | EXERCISE | TOOL | PAGE |
|---|---|---|---|
| 1 | TARGETED PALM RELEASE | ○ | P136 |
| 2 | NECK RELEASE | ▱ | P132 |
| 3 | TARGETED CHEST RELEASE | ○ | P120 |
| 4 | TARGETED SHOULDER RELEASE | ○ | P112 |
| 5 | TARGETED MIDDLE BACK RELEASE | ○ | P108 |
| 6 | TARGETED HAMSTRINGS RELEASE | ○ | P74 |
| 7 | TARGETED GLUTEAL GROUP RELEASE | ○ | P60 |
| 8 | TARGETED QUADRICEPS RELEASE | ○ | P68 |
| 9 | TARGETED CALF RELEASE | ○ | P88 |
| 10 | TARGETED FOOT RELEASE | ○ | P95 |

# SPORTS PROGRAMS

# PRE-WORKOUT

To provide a dynamic warm-up for your muscles, a routine should include as much foam rolling as possible, in addition to challenging activation movements. Complete these exercises to loosen your muscles for an injury-free workout.

## WHAT YOU NEED

- Foam roller
- Half roller
- Yoga mat

## WHAT TO DO

- Do the exercises in order.
- Spend 30 to 45 seconds on each exercise.
- Breathe deeply and relax your muscles.
- Maintain a moderate pace for exercises 5 through 8 to accelerate your circulation.

| | EXERCISE | TOOL | PAGE |
|---|---|---|---|
| 1 | GLUTEAL GROUP RELEASE | | P58 |
| 2 | QUADRICEPS RELEASE | | P66 |
| 3 | OUTER THIGH AND HIP RELEASE | | P70 |
| 4 | SPINE RESTORATION | | P98 |
| 5 | STRAIGHT-LEG RAISE | | P40 |
| 6 | STRAIGHT-LEG GLUTEAL BRIDGE | | P64 |
| 7 | ROLLER ROLLOUT | | P26 |
| 8 | OVERHEAD SQUAT | | P44 |

### HOW IT HELPS
Warming up gently increases your heart rate to loosen joints and increase blood flow to muscles.

STRAIGHT-LEG RAISE

# POST-WORKOUT

After any kind of workout, your body needs time to slow the heart rate and maximize gains in range-of-motion of the muscles. Perform this program to restore a comfortable breathing pattern and to ensure post-workout flexibility.

## WHAT YOU NEED

- Foam roller
- Yoga mat

## WHAT TO DO

- Do the exercises in order.
- Spend 30 to 45 seconds on each exercise.
- Breathe deeply and relax your muscles.
- Repeat the program if your heart rate is still rapid after the first completion.

| EXERCISE | TOOL | PAGE |
|---|---|---|
| 1 ROLLER WALKOUT | | P28 |
| 2 SIDE-LYING RIBCAGE ROTATION | | P38 |
| 3 BIRD DOG REACH | | P30 |
| 4 HIP SWIVEL | | P32 |
| 5 HALF-KNEELING RIBCAGE ROTATION | | P36 |

ROLLER WALKOUT

# STRAIGHT-LINE SPORTS

Straight-line sports like running and skiing require core stability and healthy mobility in the ankles, hips, and thoracic spine. Complete this program to reinforce core and lower body coordination for more functional forward motion.

## WHAT YOU NEED

Massage stick
Foam roller
Chair
Yoga mat

## WHAT TO DO

- Do the exercises in order.
- Spend 30 to 45 seconds on each exercise.
- Breathe deeply and relax your muscles.
- Modify any exercise that becomes too easy, or increase your repetitions.

| | EXERCISE | TOOL | PAGE |
|---|---|---|---|
| 1 | ARCH RELEASE | | P94 |
| 2 | INNER THIGH RELEASE | | P76 |
| 3 | OUTER THIGH AND HIP RELEASE | | P70 |
| 4 | CLAMSHELL HIP ROTATION | | P56 |
| 5 | STRAIGHT-LEG RAISE | | P40 |
| 6 | ROLLER WALKOUT | | P28 |
| 7 | HALF-KNEELING CORE ROTATION | | P36 |
| 8 | PLANK PROGRESSIONS | | P24 |

HALF-KNEELING CORE ROTATION

# ROTATIONAL SPORTS

Sports like baseball, tennis, and golf demand the ability to coordinate torso rotation with lower body movement. Do these exercises to improve your balance and stability during movements like swinging a racquet.

## WHAT YOU NEED

- Lacrosse ball
- Foam roller
- Half roller
- Yoga mat

## WHAT TO DO

- Do the exercises in order.
- Spend 30 to 45 seconds on each exercise.
- Breathe deeply and lengthen your torso.
- Remove your shoes for the first exercise to improve balance for the whole program.

| | EXERCISE | TOOL | PAGE |
|---|---|---|---|
| 1 | TARGETED FOOT RELEASE | | P95 |
| 2 | SPINE RESTORATION | | P98 |
| 3 | LATS RELEASE | | P122 |
| 4 | SPIRAL CALF RAISE | | P90 |
| 5 | BIRD DOG REACH | | P30 |
| 6 | HIP SWIVEL | | P32 |
| 7 | PLANK PROGRESSIONS | | P24 |
| 8 | ROTATIONAL LUNGE | | P46 |

ROTATIONAL LUNGE

**TIP**
For healthy rotation during your sport, think about the motion occurring in your chest, not your lumbar spine.

# OVERHEAD SPORTS

Overhead sports like swimming, baseball, and volleyball require strong and flexible shoulder joints and upper body muscles to safely perform the reaching movements. Do these exercises to improve the mobility of your shoulder complex.

## WHAT YOU NEED

- Foam roller
- Half roller
- Yoga mat

## WHAT TO DO

- Do the exercises in order.
- Spend 30 to 45 seconds on each exercise.
- Breathe deeply and relax your muscles.
- Perform additional repetitions if an exercise becomes too easy.

| EXERCISE | TOOL | PAGE |
|----------|------|------|
| 1 SPINE RESTORATION | | P98 |
| 2 LATS RELEASE | | P122 |
| 3 MIDDLE BACK ACTIVATION | | P110 |
| 4 SHOULDER BLADE MOBILIZATION | | P116 |
| 5 FRONT SHOULDER RELEASE | | P115 |
| 6 FOREARM WALL SLIDE | | P130 |
| 7 ROLLER ROLLOUT | | P26 |
| 8 OVERHEAD SQUAT | | P44 |

OVERHEAD SQUAT

# INDEX

## ABOUT THE AUTHOR

Sam Woodworth is a personal trainer with a degree in Exercise Science from Ball State University. He is a certified Level 2 Functional Movement Systems Professional and a Level 2 EBFA Barefoot Training Specialist. Sam strives to keep people pain-free by identifying occupational and recreational obstacles and ensuring they have the tools for healthy movement. As a trainer, Sam uses foam rollers and other myofascial release equipment with clients to improve mobility and stability, ease pain, and promote recovery. Contact Sam for further information and answers to your questions about functional movement by visiting his website: samwoodworth-trainer.com.

## ACKNOWLEDGMENTS

First and foremost, thank you to my mom, Karen Woodworth. You are without a doubt the most influential person in my life, and I owe everything to your hard work and unconditional love. Thank you also to Art Brock and Teresa Rogers for giving me the opportunity six years ago to help others and to come into my own as I do what I love. Lastly, thank you to my editor, Ann Barton: you've undoubtedly changed my life for the better by giving me this opportunity to positively affect people's lives on a big scale. Thank you, all!

## PUBLISHER'S ACKNOWLEDGMENTS

The publisher would like to thank Sam Woodworth, Niki Waddell, Cort Post, and Olga Alkhutova for their modeling talent.

**Publisher:** Mike Sanders
**Associate Publisher:** Billy Fields
**Acquisitions Editor:** Ann Barton
**Development Editor:** Alexandra Elliott
**Cover Designer:** Harriet Yeomans
**Book Designer:** XAB Design
**Photographer:** Matt Bowen
**Prepress Technician:** Brian Massey
**Proofreader:** Amy Borrelli
**Indexer:** Brad Herriman

First American Edition, 2016
Published in the United States by DK Publishing
6081 E. 82nd Street, Indianapolis, Indiana 46250

Published in the United States by Dorling Kindersley Limited.

ISBN: 978-1-4654-5350-1

Library of Congress Catalog Number: 2016938284

**Note:** This publication contains the opinions and ideas of its author(s). It is intended to provide helpful and informative material on the subject matter covered. It is sold with the understanding that the author(s) and publisher are not engaged in rendering professional services in the book. If the reader requires personal assistance or advice, a competent professional should be consulted. The author(s) and publisher specifically disclaim any responsibility for any liability, loss, or risk, personal or otherwise, which is incurred as a consequence, directly or indirectly, of the use and application of any of the contents of this book.

**Trademarks:** All terms mentioned in this book that are known to be or are suspected of being trademarks or service marks have been appropriately capitalized. Alpha Books, DK, and Penguin Random House LLC cannot attest to the accuracy of this information. Use of a term in this book should not be regarded as affecting the validity of any trademark or service mark.

DK books are available at special discounts when purchased in bulk for sales promotions, premiums, fund-raising, or educational use. For details, contact: DK Publishing Special Markets, 345 Hudson Street, New York, New York 10014 or SpecialSales@dk.com.

Printed and bound in China

All images © Dorling Kindersley Limited
For further information see: www.dkimages.com

**www.dk.com**

A WORLD OF IDEAS:
**SEE ALL THERE IS TO KNOW**